THE
LIVING
HEART

THE LIVING HEART

Michael DeBakey, M.D.

and

Antonio Gotto, M.D.

Illustrated by
Herbert R. Smith

DAVID McKAY COMPANY, INC.
New York

Library of Congress Cataloging in Publication Data

DeBakey, Michael Ellis,   1908-
  The living heart.

  Includes index.
  1. Cardiovascular system—Diseases. 2. Cardio-
vascular system.   I. Gotto, Antonio, joint author.
II. Title. [DNLM: 1. Cardiovascular system—Popular
works. 2. Cardiovascular diseases—Popular works.
WG113 D286L]
RC672.D4   616.1   76-47013
ISBN 0-679-50575-X

10 9 8 7 6 5 4

MANUFACTURED   IN   THE   UNITED   STATES   OF   AMERICA

Designed by C.R. Bloodgood

FOREWORD

THIS book by Dr. Michael DeBakey and Dr. Antonio Gotto provides the layman with a concise, authoritative guide to the cardiovascular system, how it functions and what can go wrong and why. It describes what can be done to prevent, contain or repair damage to the heart or blood vessels resulting from various disease processes.

The authors are eminently qualified to write this book. Dr. DeBakey, a premier cardiovascular surgeon, has pioneered the development of new methods and devices for the diagnosis and treatment of heart disease, including a variety of mechanical devices to aid failing hearts. He was among the first physicians to warn the public of the health hazards of cigarette smoking. As a medical statesman, he has had a profound influence over the years on the development of national health policy and federal biomedical research programs.

Dr. Gotto has performed important research on fats in the blood, the way they are metabolized and their role in the development of coronary heart

v

disease. This work has resulted in valuable insights which physicians and their patients can use to protect their hearts.

Drs. DeBakey and Gotto have established a National Heart and Blood Vessel Research and Demonstration Center at Baylor College of Medicine, the first such comprehensive center founded in the United States. Its major purpose is to demonstrate to other institutions and communities the best and quickest way to introduce new knowledge about the diagnosis and treatment of heart disease into medical practice. In all its programs, the center emphasizes prevention through public health education and motivation.

The book reflects the philosophy that prevention is the only way to significantly reduce death and sickness from heart disease and that prevention requires an informed and motivated public. Had it been written twenty-five years ago, most of the chapters would be considerably shorter, or missing altogether. For more has been learned during the past twenty-five years about the cardiovascular system and the diseases that afflict it than during all previous years of medical history. Similarly, a great many of the techniques now in widespread use for the prevention, diagnosis and relief of cardiovascular disorders were developed or perfected during this period.

For example, twenty-five years ago only a few of the thirty-five recognized types of congenital malformations of the heart and great vessels could be corrected or palliated by surgery. Today, the great majority of these cardiac birth defects can be alleviated, including all of the most common types. The percentage of patients cured or greatly improved by surgery has continued to rise, while the risk that inevitably attends any open-heart procedure has continued to decrease.

The past twenty-five years have seen similar strides in the development of "spare parts," or prosthetic devices for the heart and blood vessels. These include synthetic blood vessels, a variety of clinically-proven artificial valves, and artificial pacemakers for patients whose hearts can't be trusted to beat regularly unaided. Dr. DeBakey, in fact, pioneered the development of a technique in which surgeons use patches, or lengths of synthetic blood vessels, to remove local obstructions from the small but vital arteries which nourish the heart, kidneys and brain. Collectively, these techniques have saved many thousands of lives, and bettered the quality of life for countless others, by relief of pain and improvement of circulation.

Research and development is continuing on devices and techniques to provide temporary assistance to impaired, failing hearts while they mend, and on total artificial replacements for hearts damaged beyond repair.

Most of the drugs currently used to control high blood pressure were not available twenty-five years ago. Among the limited number that were, most produced such severe side effects that many patients preferred to take their chances with the disease. Today, a wide variety of effective drugs permit adequate control of hypertension without undue hardship on the patient.

These agents can dramatically reduce the threat of stroke, heart failure and kidney failure—the consequences of uncontrolled hypertension.

Twenty-five years ago, coronary heart disease and its complications—heart attacks, angina pectoris, and sudden cardiac death—were the leading causes of disability and death in America. They still are. But today, the heart-attack patient who reaches the hospital alive has a much better chance of surviving thanks to intensive coronary care units providing close medical supervision, continuous patient monitoring, improved emergency drugs and resuscitation procedures, and an aggressive approach to the treatment of heart-rhythm disturbances and other potentially dangerous complications. Surgery is now used to improve the blood supply to the hearts of an estimated 25,000 patients a year with angina pectoris, very often resulting in a striking relief of symptoms.

But perhaps of greatest importance for the future is what we have learned about the role high blood fats, hypertension, and smoking play in the development of premature coronary heart disease. We now know that reducing or eliminating these and other conditions can significantly decrease the chances of heart attack, and lessen the national toll of sickness and death from cardiovascular diseases.

Except for coronary heart disease, death rates have declined steadily in most cardiovascular-disease categories over the past twenty-five years. Reductions have been most dramatic for infectious heart diseases, hypertension, and rheumatic heart disease. And even for coronary heart disease, mortality rates that had been rising relentlessly for decades flattened out during the sixties and now are declining a bit.

Dr. DeBakey's and Dr. Gotto's message is clear: Biomedical research has afforded physicians great knowledge and capability. But if we are serious about preventing premature death and disability from heart disease, we must recognize that the potential for good health rests within ourselves, and then act accordingly.

Theodore Cooper, M.D.,
Assistant Secretary for Health,
Department of Health, Education, and Welfare
May 1976

PREFACE

THROUGHOUT the Western world, and now even in Russia and China, heart disease has become the most common cause of death, accounting for more deaths than all other diseases combined. In the United States more than one million people die annually from cardiovascular disease. It is estimated that more than 30 million people suffer from some form of heart disease, which causes an economic drain of more than $40 billion on the nation in cost of treatment and loss of productivity. This disease is, therefore, one of great magnitude and gravity, and requires an organized, concerted effort directed toward its control and ultimate eradication.

Although the cause of most forms of cardiovascular disease, including, particularly, arteriosclerosis and atherosclerosis (hardening of the arteries), which are by far the most common, remains obscure, rapid strides have recently been made toward developing a better understanding of the insidious abnormal changes in the arterial wall, more precise diagnostic methods, and more effective treatment. Indeed, greater advances have been made in the cardiovascular field during the past several decades than in all previous recorded medical history. These noteworthy achievements have largely been made possible due to the rapid expansion and intensification of research programs that resulted from a simultaneous increase in financial support. These advances can virtually be charted in relation to this increased aid, beginning with the establishment of the National Heart Institute (now known as the National Heart, Lung and Blood Institute) in 1948. This typically American effort of combining private enterprise with federal support in the field of medical research represents one of the most successful collaborative programs ever launched. A great deal of credit must be given to the imaginative members of Congress and the executive branch of our government, who not only responded to public interest in medical research, but also provided the leadership needed to further this truly humanitarian endeavor.

In addition to the development of strikingly more effective diagnostic and therapeutic methods, strong evidence is accumulating which indicates a reversal in the increasing mortality rate from cardiovascular disease. Thus, the death rates for stroke and rheumatic heart disease, particularly among persons younger than sixty-five, have shown impressive reductions of about 20 percent and 30 percent, respectively. The mortality rate from hypertension has been lowered even more, and an estimated 14,000 Americans who would have died of coronary arterial disease last year are alive today. It is hoped that this achievement will provide the impetus to further strengthen and accelerate medical research until the remaining medical problems are resolved.

The commonly used term heart disease is so ill-defined and all-encompassing as to be confusing, misleading, and, too often, unnecessarily alarming. Actually, many different types of diseases of the heart and blood vessels are included in the medical term cardiovascular disease. And more than three-fourths of all kinds of heart disease are diseases of the major arteries, not of the heart. They are generally due to atherosclerosis, which produces changes in the arterial wall that block blood flow through the vessel or weaken the wall and result in its ballooning out. This aneurysm may ultimately rupture and cause fatal internal hemorrhage. Thus, the "heart attack," is basically caused by arteriosclerosis or atherosclerosis of the coronary arteries which supply blood to the heart. The resulting blockage of these arteries diminishes the supply of blood to the heart muscles, thus causing sufficient damage to produce a "heart attack." The same type of disease in the arteries to the brain may bring on a stroke; in the arteries in the legs it can cause difficulty in walking and even gangrene. Aneurysms often affect the aorta and major large arteries.

Through intensive experimental and clinical investigation, considerable progress has been made toward better understanding the nature of arteriosclerosis, commonly referred to as "hardening of the arteries." Atherosclerosis is a specific type of arteriosclerosis in which fat, or lipid, is deposited initially in the innermost layer of the arterial wall. It is now known that both aneurysmal and occlusive diseases show distinctive clinical patterns in extent, location, and rate of progress. The earlier prevailing belief that arteriosclerosis was a degenerative, diffuse disease has been largely dispelled. It is now established that the disease often tends to be well localized to certain parts of the arterial system, with relatively normal areas immediately above and below the diseased segment. This concept is the basis for effective surgical treatment. Since the disease is often localized, it may be possible to remove a diseased segment and replace it with a synthetic arterial graft; simply cut out the obstructing material (endarterectomy), or bypass the diseased segment by attaching a synthetic arterial graft above and below the blockage to shunt blood around it. By using arteriography, which permits x-ray visualization of the arteries, the precise site and extent of the diseased segment can be determined.

Also of great importance is the fact that the rate of development of arteriosclerosis varies considerably in different patients. In some, for example, the disease tends to progress slowly over a period of as much as ten to twenty years, whereas in others it tends to develop rapidly, often causing serious or fatal consequences within a few years. Between these two extremes are the mild to moderate rates of development, which, in some instances, are characterized by alternating periods of stability and renewed progression. The reason why various patterns of the disease differ in extent, localization, and rate of progression is unknown, and hopefully, further research will determine this in the near future.

Certain forms of heart disease are diseases of the heart itself. These may be congenital defects, which are due to "something going wrong" during embryologic development, or they may be acquired diseases, due to certain infections, such as rheumatic fever, resulting in valvular heart disease, or they can be of an undetermined cause.

Despite the tremendous advances that have been made, there are still some forms of heart disease for which little or nothing can be done, but there are now methods of medical and surgical treatment that enable most patients to resume a normal life, and some even to be considered cured. Thus, a generation ago, a child with congenital heart disease was doomed to an early death, whereas today about 80% of these children can be cured by surgery and look forward to living a normal life. Many forms of acquired heart disease, including arteriosclerotic or atherosclerotic disease, are now amenable to effective medical and surgical treatment. The diagnosis of heart disease, which once had the alarming connotation of sealing the fate of the victim to a life of suffering, disability and early death, now has a much more optimistic prognosis.

This book was written to provide the layman with a better understanding of heart disease, particularly to define and characterize the many different forms of disease of the heart and blood vessels, to indicate what can be done about it, and to suggest what a person can do to help prevent its development. It was not our intent to prepare a comprehensive treatise or textbook of cardiovascular disease. The greatest emphasis is on the more common forms of the disease and those for which the most can be done from the point of view of treatment and prevention. Selection of historical aspects was partly based on relevance of the material to an understanding of current concepts of cardiovascular problems. To be sure, much of this information may be obtained from your physician, who must be relied upon to determine the final diagnosis and treatment. It is hoped, however, that this book will supplement your physician's judgment and will provide a better understanding of his or her recommendations. We are convinced that an informed public is much more capable of facing and resolving problems, and hope that this book will provide some enlightenment about heart disease.

We would like to express our grateful appreciation to Dr. Hebbel Hoff, Professor of Physiology, Baylor College of Medicine, for his valuable assistance in the preparation of the material on the historical and physiological aspects of the text, and to Dr. Kinsman A. Wright, Assistant Professor of Medicine, Baylor College of Medicine, for his helpful suggestions concerning the chapter on artificial cardiac pacemakers. We also wish to acknowledge Mr. Gerald Astor for his valuable help in reviewing and preparing material which provides the basis for certain sections of the text. Finally, we would like to express our gratitude to Mr. Herbert Smith for the lucid illustrations which not only supplement the text, but also provide the reader with a much better understanding of it.

> Michael E. DeBakey, M.D.
> Antonio M. Gotto, Jr., M.D., Ph.D.
> June 1976

CONTENTS

THE
LIVING
HEART

1

EARLY

KNOWLEDGE

THE organs of the body might be likened to a series of working engines. For example, the heart, which is linked to all of them, is a two-stage stroke pump. The liver and the intestines refine the fuels used by the body's engines. The kidneys, lungs, bowels and liver are sanitation units, disposing of potential pollutants, wastes or the ashes left after fuel is consumed. From the air, the lungs mine oxygen, a vital component required by any internal combustion engine. The central nervous system serves as a computer, programming the work demanded by the body's engines and monitoring the levels of performance. The human body is not quite a self-contained apparatus—outside supplies of food, oxygen and water must be brought in to stoke the machinery. But an ecological efficiency characterizes bodily functions. Blood cells, for example, nourish tissues that, in turn, help produce new blood cells. The heart keeps the digestive organs alive and these, in turn, reciprocate. Worn out cells are broken down, some elements are salvaged and recycled back into the system. For this reason, too, in any consideration of "heart disease," it is important to realize that the heart itself is but a link in a complex machine known as the cardiovascular system (Figure 1) and is itself a part of the infinitely more complex microcosm constituting the whole individual.

To the ancients, this chain of organs beneath the skin posed as much of a mystery as the world that lay beyond a few days' journey from their homeland. One of the first scholars to clarify knowledge about the structure of the heart and other organs was the Alexandrian physician Erasistratus, who recorded his observations of dissected animals and humans 2,300 years ago. To be sure, the cave paintings made by our ancestors some 20,000 years ago depicted the heart in its proper position on outlines of the bison and elephants they hunted; its shape was much like the stylized heart we see today on St. Valentine's Day. Undoubtedly, they had an idea of its vital nature. It was not, however, until the time of the Greeks (around the fifth century B.C.) that their more enlightened religious and philosophical outlook permitted anatomical studies to be made on man himself.

Prior to the time of the Greeks, disease was more often attributed to supernatural rather than to natural causes. Indeed, during the early years of Greek history, medical care was often provided by the priest who specialized as a healer. Much earlier than this, treatment by surgery and the treatment of "disease" became separated because an understanding of the supernatural was not needed to explain the occurrence of a simple wound. This distinction between surgeons and physicians continued for many hundreds of years, and we find the barber-surgeon active during the Middle Ages and the Renaissance. Hippocrates, the great Greek physician, knew much about wound surgery, had a keen eye for physical diagnosis and compiled the first descriptions of many ailments we know today. He recognized that diseases run a course, and ascribed sickness to an imbalance in the "humours" or juices of the body. Even today we talk of a "good humored" or a "bilious" person.

Probably because the Egyptians had earlier practiced the art of embalming and had removed some of the body's organs, Erasistratus was able to study some organs rather thoroughly. He discovered three pathways— *veins, arteries* and *nerves**—extending throughout the body. He also described the appearance of the heart and its valves quite accurately. But unable to grasp the notion of muscular tissue, Erasistratus decided the heart itself consisted of a conjunction of veins, arteries and nerves. Obedient to the dogma of his predecessors, Erasistratus accepted the theory that the arteries contained an air, or spirit or soul, called "pneuma," which was replenished by breathing. This pneuma was supposed to enter the body through the route of the nose, throat and lungs. According to Erasistratus and other physicians of the time, the veins contained blood which flowed along these pathways to feed the rest of the body. To Erasistratus, blood was found in arteries only after the surgeon cut the vessel open; as the pneuma rushed out, the blood poured into the empty space.

Erasistratus also pointed out specific changes in the organs of the dead

---

*Definitions and/or explanations of the italicized words that appear throughout the text can be found either in the surrounding copy or in the glossary at the back of the book.

which could be related to the cause of death. Four centuries later, however, the insights of Erasistratus were vastly reinforced by Galen, the great physician of the Roman Empire who was born a Greek in A.D. 130. Practicing in the Roman city of Perzmos in Asia Minor, Galen dissected the great apes and lesser animals brought to the gladiatorial ring by the roving Roman legions. He expanded anatomical knowledge enormously with his recognition of muscle as one of the substances that make up the human heart. He demonstrated that arteries held blood, not air, as Erasistratus insisted. Galen even spoke of the movement of blood, although he asserted that the fluid in the arteries ebbed and flowed with the heart's pulsation. Relying heavily on the correlation of experimental findings and careful clinical observations, Galen began to correlate function and structure. Like Erasistratus, he proposed hypotheses about the way organs of the body work, based on what he had learned from his experiments. One hypothesis concerned the relationship of the right and left ventricles, the two largest chambers of the heart. Galen hypothesized that tiny pores in the wall that separates these chambers permits blood to pass from the right side to the left from where it enters the arteries and passes throughout the body. Although he was wrong, Galen was on the right track in his suggestion that blood moved from one side of the heart to the other. He was so highly regarded as a physician that his suggestions were accepted as dogma until the time of William Harvey, who was born in 1578, 1,448 years after Galen's birth. Galen is quoted as saying "if anyone desires to become famous, all that is necessary is to accept what I have established" and "never yet have I gone astray."

Between the age of Galen and the Renaissance came a period of decline in medical knowledge, particularly in the search for new information. While scattered throughout Europe were some men who respected knowledge, they were convinced that everything had been revealed. Hence, they no longer searched for new information, and advancement of scientific and medical knowledge came to a halt. In Europe, Galen's theories, codified and made rigid, stood as the limits of information in medicine. Superstition and religion blocked autopsies of the dead. Not until the thirteenth century, at Bologna, is there any record of dissection of a human body.

Fortunately, medical scholarship did not die out. A Christian sect, the Nestorians,* were proscribed as heretics and forced to flee eastward, carrying with them the whole of the Byzantine culture, including medicine. Reestablished in Persia, the cult flourished, a great medical school was

---

*Nestorians were named after Nestorius, appointed the Patriarch of Constantinople by Emperor Theodosius in 428. Nestorius outraged the Catholic world by opposing the use of the title Mother of God for the Virgin on the grounds that while the Father begot Jesus as God, Mary bore him as a man. This view was contradicted by Cyril, Patriarch of Alexandria, and both sides appealed to Pope Celestine I. In 431 the Council of Ephesus was convened to settle the matter and the decision was made to excommunicate Nestor and his followers. Nestor was then deposed and exiled by Theodosius who ordered the consecration of a new Patriarch of Constantinople.

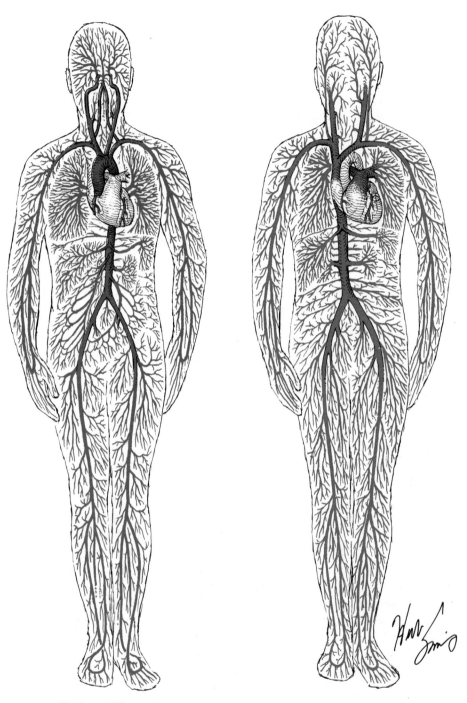

Figure 1. The cardiovascular system is one of several systems that make up the human body. The arteries carry bright red oxygenated blood from the heart to the various tissues of the body. Veins then carry the bluish deoxygenated blood back to the heart, which then pumps it through the lungs for a fresh supply of oxygen.

established, and the works of Hippocrates, Galen and many others were translated into Persian. As Persia was conquered by the Moslems, the whole of this culture was incorporated into the new Islamic culture. Great physicians founded hospitals, medical schools were established, new medical works began to appear and new diseases were described. Physicians were respected as never before. When Europe was again prepared to receive its medical culture, it was ready and waiting, preserved by cultures in the East.

The Renaissance brought a new thirst for exploration. Along with daring voyages on the high seas came a new breed of scientists peering into the mysteries of life. They soon found that the learning of the past was overly dogmatic; it had lost the very spirit of medical inquiry that gave greatness to Hippocrates and Galen; fruitless theories had been exaggerated beyond all reason. One who dared to challenge the static dogma of Galen was the itinerant Swiss physician Paracelsus, himself the son of a doctor. Success with notables brought his appointment as town physician at Basel and the right to lecture at the university. Like so many of his predecessors, Paracelsus tried to create a philosophy that might explain brith, growth and death. Out of the depths of his own experiences, he rejected the theories of Hippocrates and Galen. To scholars at the university, Paracelsus thundered, "We shall free it [medicine] from its worst errors, not by following that which those of old taught, but by our own observation of nature, confirmed by extensive practice and long experience. Who does not know that most doctors make terrible mistakes, greatly to the harm of their patients? Who does not know that this is because they cling too anxiously to the teachings of Hippocrates, Galen . . . " To demonstrate his own independence, Paracelsus made a public bonfire of his personal collection of the teachings of Galen.

In an era when the Protestant Reformation had begun to dispute the dogma and works of the Roman Catholic Church, Paracelsus decided against rebellion and remained in the Church. Nevertheless, because of his outspoken views, town authorities usually encouraged him to move on before he stayed very long, condemning him to a peripatetic existence much like the old Greek physicians. This life suited Paracelsus, however, and each town gave him something new to study and time to work on a new book perhaps, before he moved on. In one town he saw miners' disease and described an occupational disease for the first time. In another he studied the mineral springs known for their health-giving qualities and wrote, again as a first, a book on balneo-therapy. Paracelsus introduced the treatment of syphilis with mercury, the only successful therapy until Paul Ehrlich introduced the arsenicals at the beginning of the twentieth century. He also had very modern ideas about the natural care of wounds. So Paracelsus's legacy was to open the door to scientific study a crack wider; eventually most of his findings were published with their cryptic statements and self-coined words, full of hidden meanings for us to puzzle over.

In their pursuit of knowledge, Renaissance thinkers wandered from one discipline to another, their curiosity boosting them over the barriers that normally separate one field of thought from another. To the Renaissance scholar, botany, astronomy, physiology, mathematics, painting, poetry and theology were all interrelated. If this led to the well-rounded man that we praise as the shining achievement of the Renaissance, it also posed a distinct threat to his survival. For the intertwining of empirical scientific knowledge with the dogma of theology can result in serious problems.

A perfect illustration of the danger of combining scientific endeavor with theological proclamation was provided by a Spaniard, Michael Servetus (1511–1553). Geographer, mathematician, astronomer and part-time investigator of human anatomy, Servetus also showed an intense interest in religion. As a traveling scholar in Europe, Servetus proclaimed that the godsent spirit, so grandly infused by Galen into the veins and arteries of man, happened to be only air. Furthermore, in contradiction to Galen, Servetus wrote, "The communication between right and left ventricle does not, as generally believed, take place through the mid-wall of the heart, but in a wonderful way the subtle blood is conducted through a long passage from the right ventricle to the lungs where it is rendered light, becomes bright red in color and passes from the vein-like artery [arteria venosa] into the artery-like vein [vena arteriosa], whence it is finally carried . . . into the left ventricle." Servetus had offered an accurate description of the process by which blood becomes saturated with oxygen.

Unfortunately, Servetus's revelations were part of a book that attacked a variety of prevailing theological dogmas. John Calvin, the Protestant reformer, proved he could be as fiery in zeal as the Roman Catholic Inquisitors who had Servetus on their proscribed list. By order of Calvin, Servetus went to the stake along with his books. Although the scholar perished, he had succeeded in shedding an additional ray of light on the workings of the circulatory system.

The quest for knowledge, however, continued. The Flemish anatomist, Andreas Vesalius, born in Brussels in 1514 into a family of physicians, compiled a mammoth amount of anatomica, based on his own dissections and the discoveries of others. As a boy, he dissected all the animals he could find. He went to Paris at the age of eighteen to study anatomy, a field which was hampered by a fourteenth-century edict of Pope Boniface VIII, forbidding the cutting or dismemberment of dead bodies. The original intent of the edict had been to curb the practice during the Crusades of cutting off parts of the body, boiling them and preserving them until they could be taken home and buried. An unintended consequence of the edict was to impair the study of anatomy. But in Paris the Renaissance was in full swing and two great teachers, Winter of Andernach and Sylvius became Vesalius's special mentors; he performed many dissections for their classes.

Vesalius eventually obtained a medical degree in 1537. In Paris, and subsequently in Padua, he was constantly plagued by the lack of human material for dissection. But Vesalius pursued his subject with an enthusiasm that to a nonmedical person might seem to border on the morbid. One day he noticed the intact skeleton of a man hanging from the gallows. Carrion eaters had picked the body clean of flesh. Vesalius immediately secured this "perfect" specimen. In his enthusiasm, Vesalius courted the local magistrates to obtain a convenient time for executions and the right to perform dissections on the condemned. He did not hesitate at grave robbery, spiriting away the corpse of a monk's concubine and skinning it before the bereaved could find and recognize his deceased lover.

Despite the grisly nature of his efforts, Vesalius provided a monumental contribution to empirical science. Perhaps in part because of the scarcity of material, Vesalius made the most careful and detailed dissection of each body, taking voluminous notes. He incorporated this material into his book *De Humani Corporis Fabrica*, a masterpiece of anatomical scholarship (Figure 2). It constituted a major contribution to science and medicine because

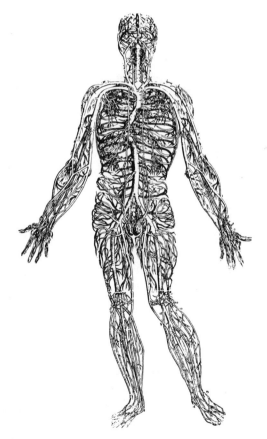

Figure 2. Sixteenth-century drawing of the cardiovascular system from the book *De Humani Corporis Fabrica* by Andreas Vesalius (Courtesy Bettmann Archive)

knowledge of anatomy of the human body is indispensable to any under-standing of normal physiology or disease processes. Vesalius discovered and exposed over two hundred errors made by Galen. Galen had written presumptuously about the anatomy of the monkey; he himself made this clear, but, in time, this fact was forgotten and Galen's anatomy was accepted as that of man. Vesalius's demonstration of the many errors in Galen's anatomy, undermined the traditional authority vested in his theories. Lectures by Vesalius were like mob scenes, with violent shouting and cheering; along with his book, they made him a controversial figure. Attacks from pro-Galenic forces, including Vesalius's former teacher, Sylvius, even-tually caused him to burn the papers and notes he was collecting for a book on medicine and pathology.

But Vesalius hewed to tradition when he discussed physiology, the science involving how the systems of the body work. He offered no coherent account of the circulation of the blood and continued to support the erroneous concept that air gets mixed into the blood in the ventricles of the heart.

Surgical treatment of disease during the Middle Ages and Renaissance was limited by the lack of adequate information about human anatomy and by the inability to control the loss of blood. Surgery was limited to very few procedures, such as pouring boiling metal or oil on wounds, excising skin tumors and removing bladder stones. The work of barber-surgeons was supervised by a physician, who did not himself practice surgery, but who had a degree.

An immediate result of the spread of the new knowledge of anatomy was a great step forward for surgery. The man personally associated with this advance was Ambroise Paré, a contemporary of Vesalius. Paré, born in 1510, had a great influence on the adoption of a humanitarian approach to the surgical treatment of battlefield wounds and the control of bleeding. Paré arrived at the Hotel Dieu, near Notre Dame, in Paris, to become a surgeon. The Hotel Dieu was used as a hospital, though it was actually an ancient hotel dating back to 660. The stench of dying and decaying flesh and the cries of the ill and near dead were overwhelming when Paré arrived. After working in this hospital for three years, Paré left to travel as personal surgeon to various aristocratic army officers and eventually to the king of France.

One of the battle surgeon's greatest challenges was the treatment of gunshot wounds. On one occasion the casualty list was so long that Paré ran out of boiling oil and only had recourse to soothing salves. Anxiously visiting the wounded the next day, Paré, expecting to find these patients either dead or dying, was surprised to see that they were in better condition and in less pain than those treated with the boiling oil. Soon he gave up the use of oil cautery entirely, and used only salves, a number of which he concocted. One employed rose oil and egg yolk; another contained two new-born puppies boiled alive, one pound of earthworms drowned in white wine, two pounds of oil of lilies, sixteen ounces of Venetian turpentine and one ounce of aqua vitae. While these recipes might not have promoted healing, the results they yielded convinced Paré that the wounds healed better if they were not cauterized with burning oil, a treatment that was not only extremely painful, but inflicted much additional damage to the tissues of the poor soldier. Paré used humanitarian arguments to support his new treatment with salves.

Another major surgical contribution of Paré's was the control of bleeding by tying off the damaged blood vessel. Paré used forceps to pick up the vessel and then secured it with a ligature. This relatively simple procedure was a giant advance in the application of surgical technique.

As further knowledge of human anatomy led to surgical advances, it gave rise to one of the most significant discoveries in the history of medicine. As a student of medicine at Padua some fifty years after Vesalius made his mark there, William Harvey (1578–1657) appropriately enough studied under Hieronymus Fabricus, then at the height of his power and fame as a professor of anatomy.

Although Fabricus accepted the whole Galenic system, he provided a key to the discovery of the circulation of the blood with his study of the valves

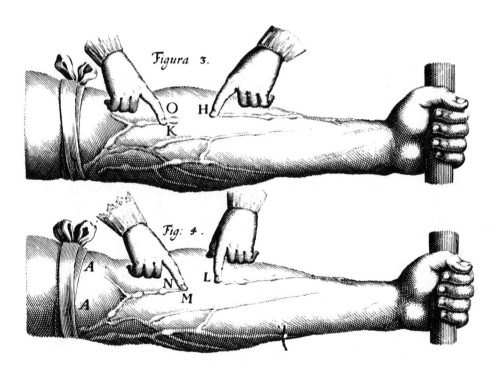

Figure 3. Classic drawing by William Harvey showing that the valves of the veins permit only one-way flow toward the heart (Courtesy Bettmann Archive)

of the veins, showing that they permitted only one-way flow toward the heart. A famous sketch by Harvey shows the effect of finger pressure upon a vein in the arm (Figure 3). When the pressure is applied, the vein collapses on the side of the pressure point closest to the heart. This demonstrates that the blood in the veins flows toward the heart.

Harvey returned from Padua to London to practice medicine, but spent most of his time studying the circulation of the blood. He was small in stature, independent in character, and worked virtually in isolation. The prevailing theory of blood circulation at the time held that there were two kinds of blood that ebbed back and forth between the arteries and veins like a tide.

Harvey's younger contemporary, the chemist and philosopher, Robert Boyle, who promulgated the laws regarding gases, once asked Harvey what inspired him to concentrate upon the heart and the circulatory system. Boyle said of the reply:

> He answer'd me that when he took notice that the Valves in the Veins of so many several Parts of the Body, were so plac'd that they gave free passage to the Blood Towards the Heart, but oppos'd the passage of the Venal blood the Contrary way: He was invited to imagine that so Provident a Cause as Nature had not so Plac'd so many Valves without Design: and no Design seem'd more probable, than that, since the Blood could not well, because of the interposing Valves, be sent by the Veins to the limbs, it should be sent through the Arteries, and return through the Veins, whose Valves did not oppose its course that way.

Harvey studied cold-blooded animals because their circulatory systems work considerably slower than those of warm-blooded ones. He observed very small shrimp, taken from the sea and the Thames River, whose transparent body walls permitted him to observe heart action while the subject lived. He also watched the earliest development of a chick heart in a hen's egg, where the tiny drop of blood actually disappears during the *systolic phase* of heart action (contraction of the heart) only to reappear slightly larger, visible to the naked eye, during the *diastolic phase* (relaxation of the heart). Harvey discovered that the function of the heart is the same in all animals, i.e. to pump blood, but that the anatomical structures of the heart and circulatory system differ in various species.

In one of his more conclusive studies, Harvey tied off the *aorta* (the main channel of blood from the heart) of a fish. He watched the aorta become bloated above the ligature as the dammed blood expanded the walls of the vessel. He then tied off the *inferior vena cava* (the main channel bringing blood back to the heart) and saw the lower half of the vessel swell with the accumulation of blood. In the aorta and its branching arteries, the blood flows from the heart to the distant parts of the body; in the veins it flows back to the heart.

A simple exercise in logic made his point about the circularity of the cardiovascular system. Harvey calculated that each beat of the heart expels about two fluid ounces of blood or 8,400 ounces per hour. Since this much blood adds up to three times the weight of an average person, the only explanation for this volume of blood was that the same six quarts of fluid were constantly circulating within the same closed system in the body.

Harvey conclusively demonstrated that blood alone travels through the arteries and veins. He quite demolished the Galenic notion that heart beat and respiration were identical twins and that air seeped into the body by means of the pores.

> For, if pulsation and respiration serve the same purposes, and if [as is commonly stated] in diastole the arteries take air into their cavities and in systole expel sooty vapours through the same pores of flesh and skin; further, if between systole and diastole they contain air, and at any given time air or spirits or sooty vapours, what answer can those holding such views make to Galen, who wrote in his book that the arteries normally contain blood and nothing but blood, certainly no spirits of air, as one can readily ascertain from his experiments, and from his arguments in that book? ... as all arteries, deep as well as cutaneous, are distended simultaneously and at equal speed, how will air be able to pass so freely and rapidly through skin, flesh and body fabric into the depths as it will through the skin alone?

Harvey's major achievement was not his destruction of the dogma of the ancients, but his conception of the heart and blood as elements within a closed, circulating system. He described the path of blood into the right side of the heart, then to the lungs, and on to the left side of the heart and the rest of the body. He concluded that the force driving the blood through the arteries comes from the pumping action of the heart, which alternately contracts and relaxes. The arteries contain no sooty vapors as air or spirits but just blood, which is returned to the heart in its rest phase through the veins. This cycle is then repeated time and time again throughout a lifetime. It remained for successors Malpigi and Leeuwenhoek, a few years later, with the aid of a new tool, the microscope, to descirbe the tiniest blood vessels, *capillaries* and *venules*, and report the final link in the system.

Harvey was able to carry out his research while physician-in-chief at Saint Bartholomew's Hospital in London. He treated patients and consulted with other physicians at the hospital one day a week. Most of the remainder of his time he devoted to research. Harvey's discoveries, published in *De Motu Cordis*, or *The Motion of the Heart*, brought him no immediate acclaim. Instead, people began to doubt his clinical ability. A contemporary reported that Harvey suffered an immediate decline in the number of patients he treated as a result of the "strange theories" he proposed. Another physician ridiculed, "Anatomy is no further necessary to a surgeon than the knowledge of the nature of wood to a carpenter or of stone to a stone cutter." Perhaps the best indication of the times is exemplified by an assignment Harvey performed six years after he described the circulation of blood. Along with six other surgeons, ten midwives and a lecturer on anatomy, Harvey served on a panel that examined four women accused of witchcraft. Stubbornly adhering to the science of empirical anatomy, Harvey found none of the extra organs or accessories with which folklore endowed witches. The women were spared the stake.

Eventually, the world did honor Harvey. He was elected president of the College of Physicians, but declined the honor. Harvey's genius explained more than the route followed by the bloodstream. He conceived of the heart, lungs and blood vessels as an interdependent system. What Harvey recognized then, holds true today—that which is labeled heart disease may not lie in the actual heart, but in other areas of the anatomy, and especially in the arterial system. And even if the problem happens to be within the heart itself, it is of little value to either the physician or the patient for the problem to be described simply as "heart disease." Cure and care depend upon a more precise diagnosis. Treatment demands knowledge of exactly what segment of the heart is injured, what function has failed, how extensive the damage is and what the threat is to the entire cardiovascular system.

With Harvey's discovery of the circulatory system, the study of anatomy was once again undertaken with a new perspective. Such studies conducted by the great surgeon and anatomist, John Hunter (1728–1793), gave rise to the field of surgical pathology, which opened the doors to knowledge about changes in the body's tissues when diseased. Here at last was a study of disease, or pathological processes, as they affect the body's organs and tissues.

There are many other milestones in medical knowledge after Harvey that are relevant to the treatment of heart disease. Among these, three are particularly important because of their great significance in surgery. The first is the development and use of anesthesia during surgery, the second is the introduction of antisepsis and asepsis to control and prevent wound infection, and the third is the advance in the knowledge of blood groups, which led to the successful introduction of *blood transfusions.* Anesthesia was first used by Dr. Crawford Williamson Long of Jefferson, Georgia. On March 30, 1842, he removed a tumor of the neck from a patient under ether anesthesia, but did not report it until 1846. The method, however, gained general acceptance and world-wide adoption following its successful demonstration by Dr. W. T. G. Morton, a Boston dentist, on a patient with a vascular tumor of the neck that was removed by Dr. John Collins Warren at the Massachusetts General Hospital on October 17, 1846.

The second important contribution, the concept of antisepsis and asepsis, was made by Joseph Lister, who as a young Glasgow surgeon recognized the significance of an earlier discovery by Louis Pasteur—the existence of bacteria. Lister reasoned that it was these minute organisms suspended in the atmosphere that were responsible for wound infection. He stated, " . . . it occurred to me that decomposition of the injured part might be avoided without excluding the air, by applying as a dressing some material capable of destroying life of the floating particles." Lister then used carbolic acid both as a carbolized dressing and as a spray to prevent infection, with considerable success. His first publication on this antiseptic method appeared in 1876, but these early reports were met with indifference and even violent opposition—mostly by his British colleagues, interestingly enough. Over the next twenty years Lister continued to work at perfecting the method, accumulating impressive evidence of its validity. Eventually it gained world-wide acceptance, thus greatly expanding the horizons of surgery.

A third major advance was the application of transfusions of whole blood to replace blood loss during surgery or after trauma or burns. Early on man had learned the danger of severe blood loss, or hemorrhage. It is a curious thing that the removal of blood from a vein, called *blood letting* or *venesection,* gained acceptance by physicians over four thousand years ago as a method of treating many forms of disease. Both Hippocrates and Galen strongly subscribed to this mode of therapy. Galen prescribed the removal of one-half to one and one-half pints of blood. In some parts of the world blood letting was used until relatively recent times. Blood transfusions, on the other hand, were not successfully utilized until the twentieth century.

To be sure, historical references to blood transfusion may be found as early as the fifteenth century, particularly after the discovery of circulation by William Harvey, in 1628. Experiments were performed on animals and, in a few cases, lamb's blood was transfused into humans. Although some success was recorded, the fatalities that occurred created much opposition and led to a legal prohibition of the procedure throughout most of Europe. Not until the nineteenth century was there a revival of interest in blood transfusion. Various investigations were carried out, mostly of a technical nature, and a few actual transfusions were performed on humans with some success, but the major obstacles of serious and even fatal complications resulting from incompatible blood hindered its adoption and widespread use.

This problem was solved by the monumental, pioneering work of Dr. K. Landsteiner, a German scientist, in 1900. In brief, Landsteiner discovered that humans can be divided into different blood groups, which are determined by the presence of certain factors on the red blood cells and in the individual's serum. Some *blood groups* are compatible with each other for purposes of transfusion, while others are not. It was not until the problems of incompatibility of blood were solved that blood transfusions could be used therapeutically.

Subsequent significant developments in this field include the use of sodium citrate to facilitate blood storage by preventing clotting, advances in blood preservation and the establishment of blood banks for matching and storing blood.

It is important to be aware of the fact that many patients with cardiovascular disease before the twentieth century were doomed, with no hope for any kind of treatment. Prior to the era of open-heart surgery, no effective treatment was available for many forms of congenital and acquired cardiac disease. There were no antibiotics for treating or preventing *bacterial endocarditis, rheumatic fever, streptococcal infections* and *cardiovascular syphilis*. Effective drug treatment for control of hypertension has only been available for about the last twenty to twenty-five years.

Today, the most prevalent form of cardiovascular disease that the physician encounters is that affecting the coronary arteries. There has been a considerable amount of disagreement as to whether the frequency of coronary disease has actually increased in the twentieth century. We suspect that it has. *Angina pectoris,* or chest pain, which is a symptom of coronary artery disease, was clearly described by William Heberden in an article entitled "Some account of a disorder of the breast," published in the Medical Transactions of the Royal College of Physicians of London in 1772. Heberden, however, did not realize that angina pectoris was associated with disease of the coronary arteries; this was discovered later by William Jenner. In 1812 John Warren wrote about angina pectoris in the first issue of the new publication, *The New England Journal of Medicine.* Some patients with angina pectoris were noted to die suddenly during an attack. The cause of death was usually given as acute indigestion. One of the most important papers ever written on this subject was published by James Herrick in the *Journal of the American Medical Association* in 1912 and was entitled "Clinical Features of Sudden Obstructions of the Coronary Arteries." Though the paper was largely ignored for several years, it clearly related obstruction of the coronary arteries to chest pain and in some instances, sudden death. Another important treatise relating angina pectoris to coronary artery disease is that of C. S. Keefer and W. H. Resnick in the *Archives of Internal Medicine* (1928) entitled "Angina Pectoris; a Syndrome Caused by Anoxemia of the Myocardium." To return to the question of whether the disease is becoming more frequent or whether it is being more accurately diagnosed, we refer to the experience in New York of Dr. Austin Flint, who wrote in 1866 that he observed only seven cases of angina pectoris in more than 150 patients with organic heart disease. It is unlikely that as astute a clinician as Flint would have failed to diagnose angina pectoris had it been as common as it is today.

2

THE BLOOD: ITS ROLE IN MAINTAINING EQUILIBRIUM IN THE BODY'S INTERNAL ENVIRONMENT

A rough metaphor provides one way of understanding the cardiovascular system. Think of the body as a continent packed with billions of people, the equivalent of the cells that make up a human being. Without adequate nourishment and sanitation, these billions will die and the continent will become lifeless. A steady flow of trucks, represented by the blood stream, carry oxygen, water and foodstuffs to the cells and haul away waste over 60,000 miles of roadway, the extent of the blood vessels in a normal adult.

The trucks with fresh loads of oxygen and foodstuffs begin their trip from the heart over a broad one-way highway, known as the aorta. Slightly smaller avenues (arteries) branch off into the countryside and these, in turn, subdivide into *arterioles*. These roadways are capable of widening themselves when some area of the body requires more supplies quickly. Finally, one

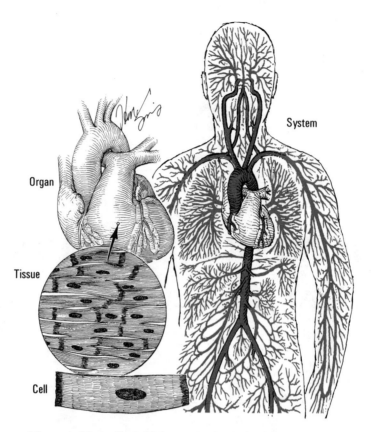

System

Organ

Tissue

Cell

Figure 4. The cells, which are the basic building blocks of the body, make up tissues such as the heart muscle. Organs, such as the heart, are made up of a number of different tissues and in turn are part of the various systems of the body, like the cardiovascular system shown here.

arrives at the capillaries, alleys so narrow that just a single vehicle, or blood cell, visible only under a powerful microscope, can squeeze through. Nestled in the spaces between cellular tissue, the capillary delivers the food and oxygen to the ultimate consumer, the cell. Simultaneously, waste is collected. Following the deliveries and collections, the blood cells enter another one-way road system, the veins, and head back to the heart. During their travels, blood cells leave nitrogen wastes in the kidneys, and carbon dioxide in the lungs for disposal. Oxygen is loaded on in the lungs and other materials are gathered from the stomach, liver, endocrine glands, *adipose tissue* and other organs. Some of these "factories" have processed supplies brought in from outside, like the food we eat.

That roughly describes the body's systems, but an understanding of the whole demands a knowledge of the parts and of the processes we call metabolism, which will be discussed in the next chapter. The basic building blocks of the entire human body are the cells, which contain various structures and chemical substances in a water solution. Combinations of cells add up to what we call tissues, while various organizations of tissue make up the organs and systems of the body (Figure 4).

The life of the cell, and therefore the continued existence of tissue and bodily organs, depends upon a continual supply of chemical substances. The bloodstream, which itself contains cellular components, delivers the required nutrients to the cells and tissues of the body. Blood must circulate twenty-four hours a day in order to sustain life. In a normal human being, this means that six quarts of blood are pumped by the heart each minute, or 2,000 gallons per day, which is over 50,000,000 gallons over a seventy-year lifetime (Figure 5). Since cells in tissues pass through their life cycle and continually break down, while new ones are constantly forming, the bloodstream also carries away the debris or nonsalvagable elements of the old cells.

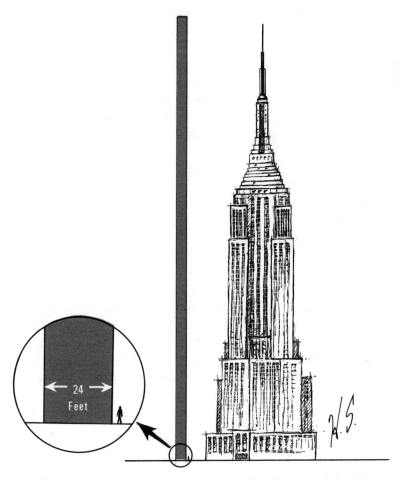

Figure 5. The fantastic volume of blood pumped by the average human heart during a person's lifetime would fill a cylinder twenty-four feet in diameter to a height taller than the Empire State Building.

The cells in the tissues of the body are located in what is called extracellular or *interstitial fluid.* Nutrients and oxygen pass into the cell from the interstitial fluid and waste products are transferred in the opposite direction from the cell to the fluid. This process is dependent on diffusion between the interstitial fluid and the blood, a process which occurs through the walls of the capillaries. The delicate regulation of fluid and salt balance between the cells and the bloodstream is called the osmotic balance. If this balance is upset, a condition known as edema occurs in which there is swelling because of an excessive accumulation of interstitial fluid.

In effect, the bloodstream can be called a river of life. In volume, the blood amounts to six quarts, or about five and one-half liters, of fluid in the average person. Approximately one-half of the volume of blood consists of cells, while the other half is a fluid called plasma. There are three types of cells in the blood: the red cells, or *erythrocytes,* white cells, or *leukocytes,* and *platelets* (Figure 6).

The erythrocytes are red blood cells which carry *hemoglobin* and support oxygen transport. They are the major cellular components of the blood and account for about 45 percent of the volume of blood in a man and 38 percent to 42 percent in a woman. Erythrocytes are flexible, elastic and concave, which is the optimal shape for promoting the exchange of gases, since the distance the gas must diffuse is decreased. The flexibility of an erythrocyte enables it to swirl through the blood vessels at considerable speed. These cells are so minute that a single cubic millimeter of blood carries about five million of them. In addition to red blood cells, there are three types of leukocytes, or white cells: polymorphonuclear leukocytes, lymphocytes, and monocytes. These cells protect the body against foreign substances and infection. A third type of blood cell, the platelet, is involved in blood clotting or coagulation, a process designed to stop bleeding when it occurs. *Plasma* is a salt and protein solution in which the blood cells are suspended. When blood clots, one of the proteins of plasma, *fibrinogen,* is converted into *fibrin,* leaving behind a fluid that is then called the *serum.* Blood clotting takes place as a consequence of the interaction of a complex series of factors in a cascade mechanism. Prothrombin, a substance which is present in normal circulation, produces a protein called *thrombin* which acts upon the protein fibrinogen to produce fibrin. The fibrin forms long threads which trap the blood cells and fluid to produce the clot. If blood escapes due to an injury to a blood vessel and comes in contact with tissue, a fibrin clot will form. In some instances, the clotting mechanism may play a role in causing heart attacks or strokes by *arterial thrombosis.*

The organs and tissues of the body add substances to the blood which are not obtained from external sources like food or air. These substances must either be manufactured or modified within the body. Examples are the chemical substances synthesized by the liver, the hormones released from the endocrine glands (including the pancreas, thyroid, pituitary, testes and ovaries) and the antibodies derived from lymphoid tissue.

The blood has a number of vital functions in addition to carrying oxygen, transporting potential energy in the form of food and providing sanitation through the elimination of waste products. The circulation helps to maintain uniform body temperature by transferring heat from warmer tissues to cooler ones.

Another important function of the blood is to defend the body against infection; antibodies, or protein globulins, react against foreign substances, while the polymorphonuclear leukocytes engulf bacteria and foreign substances. *Lymphocytes,* which are found in the bloodstream as well as in lymphoid tissue, are involved in the production of antibodies.

Plasma proteins render some of the major services performed by the blood. The plasma proteins are classified as *albumins, globulins,* and *fibrinogen,* based on their ease of precipitation or removal by various salt solutions. Associated with the protein factions are fat- or lipid-containing proteins referred to as *plasma lipoproteins,* which transport the major fats of the blood— *cholesterol, triglycerides, cholesterol esters,* and *phospholipids.* Elevations of the concentrations of these substances are associated with an increased likelihood of developing premature arteriosclerosis. Albumin serves a key role in maintaining osmotic pressure, which keeps fluid from either leaving the bloodstream too rapidly, or from building up excessively within the vascular tree.

An absolutely vital function of the blood is its transport of gases. Even when the body is at rest, it consumes oxygen. Each erythrocyte carries an oxygen-filled protein known as hemoglobin, and so it is these red blood cells that actually transport oxygen. Oxygen is not released from hemoglobin until it reaches the tissues of the body which are relatively oxygen-poor and where the environment is relatively acidic. Oxygen is then given up to the cell, and the waste product, carbon dioxide, moves from the cell into the blood to be carried to the lungs for disposal. It is mostly changes in the acidity of the environment that regulate the release of oxygen from hemoglobin. Demand for oxygen greatly increases during physical activity. Erythrocytes collect oxygen from the *alveoli,* 700 million tiny sacs in the lungs, comprising a surface area of about sixteen acres, that hold freshly inhaled air. Oxygen passes from the alveoli to the erythrocyte and associates with a molecule of hemoglobin. Simultaneously, carbon dioxide passes out into the alveoli (Figure 7).

Since the flow of blood depends upon the action of the heart, it may decrease in people with heart disease. Consequently, *anoxia,* or oxygen deficiency of the body, may occur in cases where there is an inadequate exchange of gas in the lungs, the oxygen tension is severely reduced in the air breathed, the respiratory tract is obstructed or the available hemoglobin for oxygen transport is diminished, as in carbon monoxide poisoning or as a result of drugs. Anoxia may also occur if there is impaired blood flow, hemorrhage, shock or congestive heart failure. Thus, oxygen deficiency may occur because of a decrease in the amount of oxygen carried by the blood, interference in circulation, or dysfunction in the cells. For example, cyanide poisoning results in an inability of the cell to use the oxygen supplied to it.

An interesting accommodation called acclimatization occurs when there

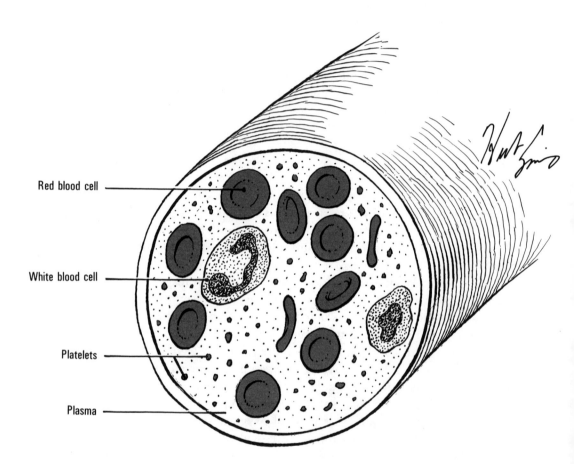

Red blood cell

White blood cell

Platelets

Plasma

Figure 6. The components of the blood

is a chronic deficiency of oxygen. This is typical of the physiological adjustment of an individual who moves to a high altitide. Initially, upon exposure to chronic anoxia at a great height, the individual experiences shortness of breath, palpitations, dizziness, weakness, impairment of mental functions, nausea and vomiting. The expression "mountain sickness" aptly describes this condition, which fortunately abates and disappears after several days. With acclimatization, there is an increase in the rate of breathing, which is probably the single most important adaptation. Depth of respiration and pulse rate also increase. The ability of the arterial blood to carry oxygen is increased by the production of additional red blood cells and hemoglobin.

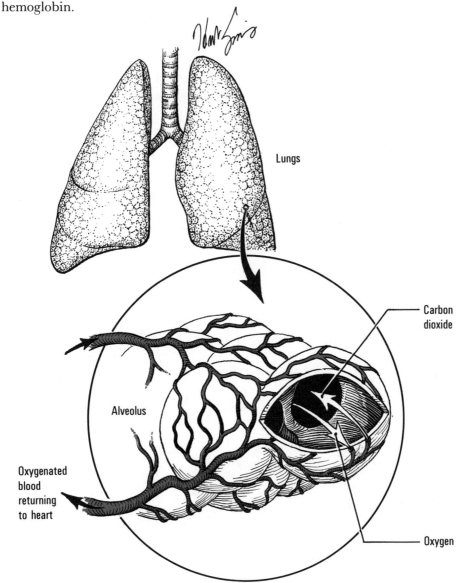

Figure 7. The alveoli of the lungs are tiny saclike structures at the terminal end of the breathing tube, where oxygen is removed from the air and taken into the blood in the surrounding blood vessels and carbon dioxide is given off.

The functioning of the bloodstream demonstrates a key concept of modern physiology, *homeostasis,* which may be summed up as an effort to preserve a relatively stable state of equilibrium in the body despite external or even internal influences. Over one hundred years ago the great physiologist, Claude Bernard, called attention to the important concept of maintenance of *le milieu interieur*. Bernard laid great stress on the importance of the blood in maintaining this state. More recently, the Boston physiologist Walter Bradford Cannon popularized this concept and named it homeostasis. We have used a number of metaphors to explain the systems of the body. Homeostasis may be compared to the operation of a greenhouse. Whatever the weather and climatic conditions beyond the glass, a certain fixed internal environment is maintained. However, it should be apparent by now that all systems in the body do not remain constant but are rather in a continual state of dynamic equilibrium. Nevertheless, variables such as body temperature, blood pressure and blood sugar concentrations are quite well regulated. If the circulation were compared to a structured society or organization, the blood would represent the transportation system, the air conditioning, the sanitation and the ventilation, and would perform these functions within a self-sealing tube.

3

METABOLISM:
CHEMICAL PROCESSES
OF THE BODY

*B*UILDING up cells usually involves forming large molecules from small ones. Conversely, the breakdown of cells is characterized by the splitting of large molecules into smaller ones. The word *metabolism,* derived from the Greek word for change, is a term used to describe the physical and chemical processes by which the living organism creates and breaks down substances and produces energy. Processes in which smaller molecules are built up into larger ones are referred to as *anabolic,* while those in which larger molecules are broken down into smaller ones are called *catabolic.* During youth, when active growth is occurring, anabolic processes predominate. In the normal mature adult, the anabolic and catabolic reactions are virtually balanced. In old age, the catabolic reactions usually predominate.

Energy to sustain the various activities of the body is derived from the foods we eat. There are three major types of foods: carbohydrates, proteins and fats. In the average American diet, approximately 20 percent of the calories come from proteins, 40 percent from fats and 40 percent from carbohydrates. Most foods must be processed in the digestive tract before

23

they can be absorbed by the body. Digestion begins in the mouth with the secretion of saliva and the chewing of food, which increases the surface area for further breakdown. Digestive enzymes secreted in the stomach and small intestine break down complex carbohydrates such as starches to form sugars. These sugars then split proteins into their constituent amino acids and *hydrolyze* dietary fat (mainly in the form of triglycerides) to fatty acids and *monoglycerides.* These end products are largely absorbed by the body from the small intestine. The water-soluble components enter the circulation via the portal vein which transports them to the liver. The water-insoluble substances, which consist mainly of triglycerides, enter the lymph and reach the circulation in the chest via lymphatic pathways (Figure 8).

In the liver, a variety of complex metabolic reactions occur. Some of the sugar, amino acids, triglycerides and phospholipids are converted into the complex carbohydrate *glycogen* which may be stored in the liver. A major storage of fat is in the adipose tissue, where the fat resides as triglyceride, until it is needed for energy. When the cells of the body require energy, it may be rapidly supplied from glucose or sugar and fatty acids. These substances see to the minute by minute energy requirements of the body's tissues. The brain has a special dependence on sugar, which it must have to survive.

Most of the chemical energy in the body, about 80 percent, is stored in the form of the fat in a lean adult, and is found in adipose tissue. On strictly a weight basis, the combustion, or burning, of fat yields more than twice as much energy as the same quantity of carbohydrate or protein. Approximately 15 percent of the fuel store of the body is protein, which cannot be combusted to provide energy because of its structural function. That is, if the protein were burned as fuel to provide energy, the muscle tissue would have to be destroyed. Thus, protein may be looked upon as an unavailable source of energy. In terms of the total energy stores of the body, carbohydrate ranks third, but, nonetheless, is more important than protein. Carbohydrate is stored in the liver and in muscle as glycogen, which is broken down by a complex sequence of chemical reactions. The net result of this adrenalin-stimulated chain of events is the breakdown of glycogen to sugar, or glucose, which can be released into the bloodstream and transported to body tissues where it is burned as fuel. Part of the normal reaction to stress involves the secretion of *adrenalin* by the adrenal gland, which causes glycogen breakdown and a rise in the level of blood sugar.

In discussions relating to diet, you may have heard some claims that calories do not count. An understanding of the concept of energy metabolism should make it clear to you that calories do, in fact, matter. During the course of an ordinary day, the normal adult uses a certain number of calories as energy. The three major factors which determine an individual's metabolic level are the degree of physical activity, the external temperature and the foods digested. In determining the basal metabolism of a subject, these three factors are controlled as far as possible. The calories expended each day may vary from 1,500 to several thousand, depending upon the degree of muscular activity. More calories are required in a cold climate than in a warm one.

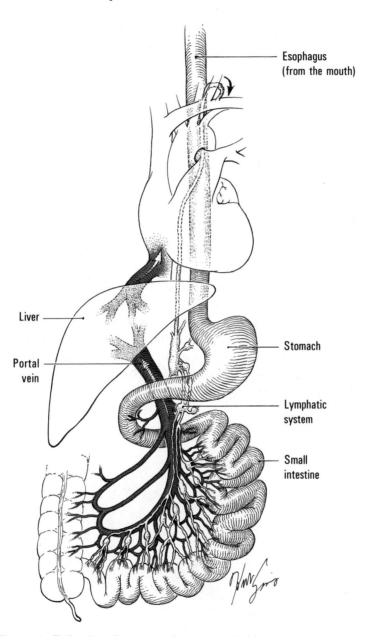

Figure 8. Following digestion, the water-soluble components of food enter the circulation by way of the portal vein, which transports them to the liver. The water-insoluble substances enter the lymphatic system and reach the circulation in the chest.

The first law of thermodynamics is one of the most important fundamental concepts in understanding metabolism. This law describes the conservation of energy and states that when a system gains or loses energy and undergoes change, the gain or loss by the system is identical to the gain or loss by the surrounding system. Thus, in a state of complete energy balance, the energy expended by an individual must equal that supplied by foodstuffs absorbed from the intestine or from food previously stored. When the calories provided by food exceed the total calories burned, the excess is stored primarily as fat in adipose tissue. Over a period of time these excess calories result in obesity.

While some tissues in the human body have a limited ability to obtain energy from *anaerobic,* or oxygenless, reactions, most energy is liberated from the combustion of foodstuffs, a phenomenon requiring oxygen. The oxygen is transported to tissues with hemoglobin, and as oxygen is released to peripheral tissues, carbon dioxide is collected in exchange. The complete combustion of foodstuffs, whether they be carbohydrate, fat or protein, produces carbon dioxide and water.

When a power plant burns coal or oil to generate electricity, there is considerable waste left over as energy is transformed into electricity. Similarly, in the body there is a residue from the chemical reactions that support physical activities. Electrical generators may get rid of their wastes in the form of smoke up a chimney or as ash hauled away by truck. The same stream that brings the necessary oxygen, glucose and other substances to the tissues also removes waste products such as carbon dioxide, which travel to the lungs and are exhaled like invisible smoke. Other molecules of waste go to the kidney, where they will be separated from the still useful components of

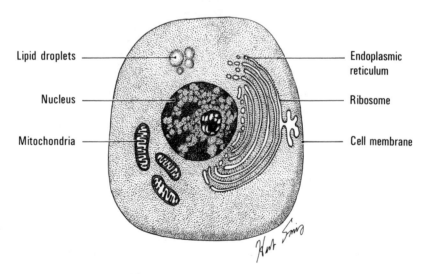

Figure 9. The structure of a cell

the blood and discharged in the urine. In addition to carbon, hydrogen and oxygen, proteins also contain the element nitrogen. In man, the nitrogen waste products are converted in the liver to the inert substance urea, which is excreted by the kidney. Certain fat-soluble substances may be excreted from the liver through the bile into the intestine and be eliminated through the stool. In speaking of the sanitation functions of the body, mention should also be made of the important role of the liver and, to a lesser extent, the lungs in breaking down foreign substances to make them less toxic. This process is called detoxification and is of great importance in the metabolism of many drugs.

The basic unit of the body is the cell (Figure 9). Within the cell are protein substances called enzymes, which catalyze, or stimulate, the anabolic and catabolic reactions. Protoplasm is the name given to the living substance which fills the cell. The nucleus of the cell is surrounded by a membrane and contains the genetic instructions that tell the cell what to do. This information is present in a coded form in a chemical substance called DNA (deoxyribonucleic acid). DNA makes up the genes of the cell, which are organized into chromosomes. Information contained in the genes tells the cell what kind of protein to make from twenty building blocks called amino acids. Thus, a liver cell makes liver proteins, a heart cell makes heart proteins and a brain cell makes brain proteins.

Instructions that tell the cell's machinery what kind of protein to make are transcribed by being coded in a special chemical message contained in another kind of nucleic acid, RNA (ribonucleic acid) (Figure 10). For this process, the DNA, which is in the nucleus, acts as a template for the formation of a molecule of RNA, which, in turn, carries a message to the protein-synthesizing apparatus outside the nucleus. As an analogy of this process, consider that the left hand is used as a mold or template to make a right hand. The two hands will be mirror images of each other. This is the way in which the genetic information is encoded and transcribed. The information is carried by the messenger RNA back to the cytoplasm, which is a term used to describe the protoplasm outside of the cell's nucleus.

Protein synthesis occurs on specialized structures called ribosomes. The ribosomes are located along a network of membranes in the cytoplasm called the endoplasmic reticulum (Figure 9). The rough endoplasmic reticulum consists of a membrane with which particles of RNA, the ribosomes, are associated. Messenger RNA carries the information that determines the character of the protein formed.

Synthesis of proteins requires energy and falls under the classification of an anabolic process. The energy which such reactions require, must be derived from chemical reactions in which foodstuffs are combusted or oxidized.

The oxidative processes that produce most of the cell's energy occur within specialized structures of the cell known as *mitochondria*, which may be likened to the power plants where coal or oil is burned to generate electricity. In man, the series of metabolic reactions is controlled by complex regulatory mechanisms which adjust them as closely as possible to the body's need at a particular time.

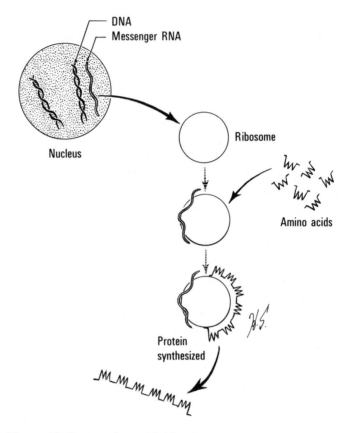

Figure 10. In protein synthesis, the messenger RNA carries information from the DNA in the nucleus to the ribosome, which assembles amino acids to produce proteins.

One type of coarse regulation is through the synthesis and breakdown of enzymes. For example, a substance which increases the synthesis of messenger RNA that codes for a particular enzyme could eventually speed up an entire sequence of chemical reactions. In contrast to coarse control of the body's chemical reactions, fine regulation may be exerted through an increase or decrease in the activity of an enzyme. For example, certain substances may interact with an enzyme at one point on the surface of the molecule and change the structure and activity of that part of the enzyme molecule that catalyzes a chemical reaction.

Many of the body's metabolic pathways are regulated by thermostatlike controls, for example, in the conversion of x to y to z, if too much z accumulates, it may shut off the sequence. By analogy, when the temperature gets too high, the thermostat shuts off the furnace and similarly, the regulatory control slows down the chain of metabolic reactions. Energy production is required for many processes within the body in addition to the synthesis of protein; for example, in the contraction of muscle in the beating of the heart, in the transmission of nerve impulses, and in the production of heat that maintains the body's temperature.

One of the most important relationships of metabolism to the cardiovascular system is the regulation of energy production and utilization during physical exercise. About 40 percent of the weight of a normal adult is made up of skeletal muscle. This mass of muscle uses about 20 percent of the oxygen consumed by the body at rest. Oxygen utilization in the burning of foodstuffs rises dramatically during periods of vigorous exercise. The combustion process is used to generate high energy phosphate *(ATP)* which is then coupled with mechanical work to support muscle contraction.

Outside of the brain, fatty acids are the main fuel used to provide energy in the resting state. During exercise, the situation changes, and the energy requirements for the muscles are provided by muscle glycogen and glucose, derived from the bloodstream, as well as by free fatty acids from the blood. During exercise, the hormones, glucagon and adrenalin, are released and stimulate the breakdown of liver glycogen with the release of glucose into the blood. Adrenalin also stimulates production of an enzyme that causes the breakdown of stored triglycerides and the release of free fatty acids into the bloodstream. Insulin levels, by contrast, are low during exercise.

During the first five to ten minutes of exercise, the glycogen within the muscle cell itself provides the major source of energy for the increased activity. The longer the exercise is continued, the more important the nutrients derived from the bloodstream become. After ten to forty minutes of exercise, the consumption of blood glucose by the muscle cell increases dramatically. After forty minutes, at least three-quarters of the carbohydrate used by the muscle cell comes from the blood sugar. Consumption of blood sugar by the muscle continues to rise for one and one-half to three hours, after which time it begins to fall off. During this period, the combustion of free fatty acids derived from the blood also increases. After four hours of exercise, the relative contribution of free fatty acids as compared to carbohydrate as a fuel source has practically doubled. Thus, the supply of fuel to meet the demands of exercise on skeletal muscle may be looked upon as occurring in three phases. The use of intracellular glycogen predominates in the early phase, blood sugar in the middle phase and the blood's free fatty acids in the last phase. It is an interesting but unexplained observation that the depletion of the intracellular muscle glycogen occurs at the same time as physical exhaustion.

During mild exercise for short periods of time, the concentration of blood sugar does not change significantly. If exercise is continued beyond one and one-half hours, the concentration of blood sugar falls by 10 to 40 milligrams percent, but only very rarely does the concentration fall below 40 milligrams percent, which is the level used to define hypoglycemia (low blood sugar). The liver is virtually the sole source of blood sugar outside of the diet. Under normal resting conditions, about three-quarters of the sugar is formed by the breakdown of glycogen, while the other one-fourth is derived from noncarbohydrate sources. This process of synthesis of glucose from noncarbohydrates is called gluconeogenesis. After exercising for more than forty minutes, the liver stores of glycogen become increasingly depleted and the liver relies more and more on gluconeogenesis for the blood sugar necessary to support the metabolic demands of the exercising muscle.

Whereas during exercise blood is preferentially shunted to the exercising limb or muscle bed, after the activity is over the blood flow is redistributed from these muscles to the abdominal organs. Now the replenishment of both liver and muscle glycogen stores begins. Anabolic reactions start to supersede the previous catabolic ones as the body prepares itself again for the challenge of a "flight and fright" stress.

4

THE
HEART AND
HOW IT WORKS

*L*OOK at your fist and you'll see an approximation of the actual size of your heart. In appearance, it more closely resembles a thick cone than the conventional valentine representation. A normal adult heart weighs about eleven ounces, although in a highly trained athlete it may be as much as a pound. This center of the cardiovascular system sits between the lungs, with its top tilted toward the right side of the body (Figure 11). Most of the heart consists of muscle, known in medical terms as the *myocardium.* Actually, this muscle is sandwiched between two thin protective layers: the *epicardium* (the outer layer) and the *endocardium* (the inner layer). The interior of the heart harbors two pairs of hollow chambers. We refer to these chambers as the right and left sides of the heart, but in point of fact the right side is located almost in front of the left side if one looks at the heart head on. Each pair contains a small antechamber—an *atrium,* or *auricle*—and a larger section called a *ventricle.*

Let us follow the circulation cycle beginning in the right atrium (Figure 12). Blood that has completed its mission of delivering oxygen and nutrition to the rest of the body empties into the right atrium from two large veins, the *inferior vena cava* and the *superior vena cava*. The former collects its cargo from the area of the body below the heart, the latter from above the heart.

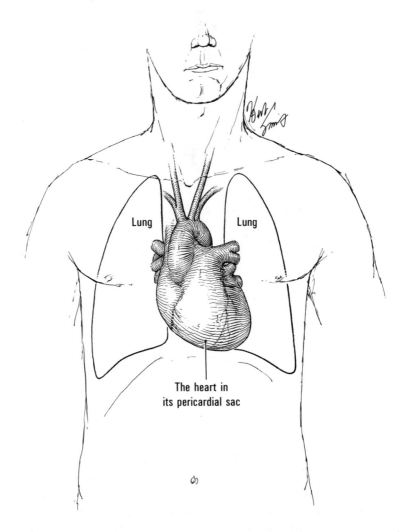

Figure 11. Relative position of the heart in the pericardial sac in the chest

Inside the top of the right atrium sits a small bundle of muscle fibers and nerves. This is the *sinoatrial node,* or *pacemaker,* (Figure 13), and at regular intervals an electrical impulse shoots out from the sinoatrial node. That charge causes the muscles of the right atrium to contract in a wavelike motion from top to bottom. The squeeze of muscle fibers exerts pressure on the blood in the atrium and the fluid seeks an outlet. Between the atrium and a much larger chamber, the right ventricle, lies the sought-for door, the

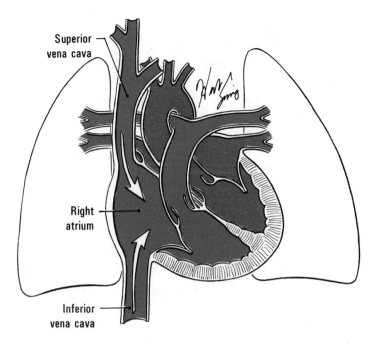

Figure 12. Deoxygenated blood from the veins of the body enters the right atrium through the superior and inferior venae cavae.

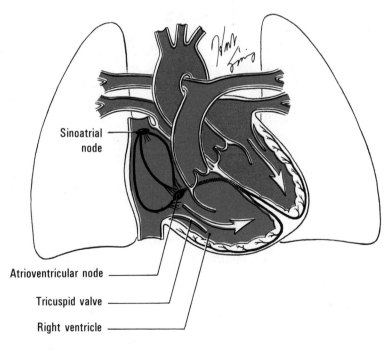

Figure 13. Normal pacemaker and conduction system

tricuspid valve, a one-way opening named for the three leaves of tissue that form it. Pressure forces the valve open and blood pours into the right ventricle. Harvey noted, " . . . if . . . with the auricle alone beating, you cut off the apex of the heart with a pair of scissors, you will see the blood flow out from the wound with each beat of the auricle. You will thus realize that the blood gets into the ventricles not through any pull exerted by the distended heart, but through the driving force exerted by the beat of the auricles."

Just as the right ventricle fills with blood, an electrical impulse fired by the sinoatrial node reaches the *atrioventricular node* (Figure 13). This is another bundle of muscle and nerves, located in the wall or septum between the two ventricles. The atrioventricular node, triggered by the charge from the sinoatrial node, passes the shock wave along two routes that quickly stimulate the rest of the heart's muscle.

The muscles of the right ventricle contract, but as the blood seeks to return to the opening from which it came, the tricuspid valve shuts when pressure in the right ventricle exceeds that in the right atrium. Since the tricuspid valve opens only one way, there can be no return of blood from the right ventricle to the right atrium. Within the right ventricle, mounting pressure forces the trapped blood to find an escape route. As the pressure in the right ventricle becomes greater than that in the *pulmonary artery,* the *pulmonary valve* is pushed open to expose a hoselike tube that divides into left and right branches leading to the two lungs (Figure 14). Passing through the branches of the pulmonary artery, the blood eventually comes in contact with the alveoli which hold oxygen inhaled through the mouth and nose.

The freshly oxygenated blood, bright crimson as a result of the infusion of oxygen, drains into a pair of pulmonary veins that lead out of each lung. These veins, like the inferior and superior vena cava, empty into another chamber of the heart, the left atrium, which is slightly larger than its right-sided colleague (Figure 14).

The electrical impulse that initiated squeezing of the muscles of the right side of the heart almost simultaneously energizes the left side, beginning with the left atrium. The contraction forces the blood in the left atrium to seek an outlet, but the route from the veins is again one way. Pressure forces open a two-leafed valve, called the *mitral valve,* and oxygenated blood enters into the largest chamber of the heart, the left ventricle. Now the rolling wave of muscular contraction begins to compress the left ventricle. The mitral valve shuts to prevent blood from returning to the atrium. The only escape is through a valve that leads to the aorta, the main artery, or pathway, of the cardiovascular system. Oxygenated blood is now on its journey to the farthest reaches of the body, bearing life-supporting supplies for the cells.

Actually, the entire process of blood filling and emptying the heart lasts less than a second. The contraction phase is called *systole,* while the relaxation period, when blood fills the atria and the ventricles, is known as *diastole* (Figure 15). Said the observant Harvey, "Those two movements, one of the auricles and the other of the ventricles, occur successively, but so harmoniously and rhythmically that both [appear to] happen together and only one movement can be seen, especially in warmer animals in rapid movement."

The action of the heart produces sounds, and long before the perfection of *electrocardiography,* doctors examined patients by means of techniques which came under the headings of percussion (tapping) and auscultation (listening). Even the school of Hippocrates described a cacophony of noises within the chests of patients. "It bubbles like boiling vinegar" or "it creaks like a new leather strap." In the eighteenth century, Leopold Auenbrugger, the son of an Austrian innkeeper, drew his inspiration from the practice of tradesmen like his father who tapped wine vats to determine the level of the contents. Auenbrugger began tapping humans, starting with himself, testing all parts of his body and then experimenting on corpses. Auenbrugger managed to distinguish between the sounds due to fluid in the chest, enlargement of the heart or thickening of the lungs. In 1761 he published these results. He observed, for example, that upon striking the thorax or chest "the sound thus elicited from the healthy chest resembles the stifled sound of a drum covered with a thick woollen cloth or other envelope." He also cataloged the many dismal sounds of chest ailments.

Auenbrugger became so discouraged by the scorn heaped upon him that he shifted his public interest to music but quietly pursued further study of percussion. Some forty years later, a French physician, Jean Nicolas Corvisart, took command of Napoleon's medical corps and adopted the technique of percussion. When Napoleon's well-renowned chief doctor advised tapping, all of Gaul's healers listened. Doctors even began to take the use of sound as a means of diagnosis a step further; they listened to the heart with an ear on the chest.

Prudery, fashion and anatomy all conspired against this form of study. Modest female patients did not dare undress before a doctor. Coarse fabrics and thick layers of undergarments muffled any sounds that might reach the discreet ear of a physician. Obesity, a common ailment among the well-to-do, the class most likely to procure the services of a doctor, made listening difficult as well. Poor hygiene also contributed to the unpleasantness of auscultation.

All of these obstacles to diagnosis through listening faced a youthful French doctor, René Laënnec, in 1816. As a doctor at Paris's Necker Hospital, he started to walk home one day while pondering what to do about a plump seventeen-year-old patient. When he passed through a restoration project in the Louvre, he noticed some children playing among the building materials. In a happy accident of discovery, he saw one boy put his ear to the end of a piece of lumber while another youngster thumped the opposite end. Immediately, Laënnec recalled the well-known acoustic phenomenon and walked back to the hospital. He seized the nearest magazine, and rolled it into a cylinder for the first use of what we know today as a stethoscope (from

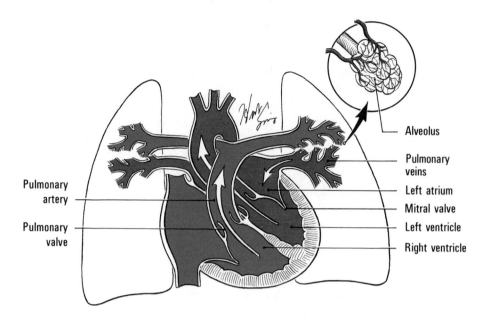

Alveolus

Pulmonary veins

Left atrium

Mitral valve

Left ventricle

Right ventricle

Pulmonary artery

Pulmonary valve

Figure 14. From the right ventricle blood is pumped through the pulmonary artery into the lungs, where it is oxygenated in the alveoli. The blood returns from the lungs through the pulmonary veins into the left atrium. After passing through the mitral valve, it is then pumped out of the left ventricle into the aorta and the arteries of the body.

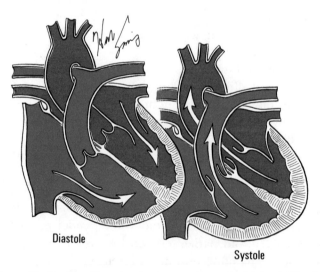

Diastole

Systole

Figure 15. During diastole, the heart relaxes and blood fills the atria and ventricles. During systole, the ventricles contract and drive the blood from the right ventricle into the lungs and from the left ventricle into the aorta and its branching arteries throughout the body.

the Greek *stethos*, chest, and the French *scope*, explore). Laënnec later refined the instrument from a paper cylinder to a wooden tube.

Laënnec embarked on an intensive research project on auscultation. At first, publication of his results brought either indifference or opposition. However, gradually the technique gained adherents. In Austria-Hungary, Laënnec's text fascinated medical student Joseph Skoda, who became such an ardent convert to the stethoscope that he took an unpaid job as an underdoctor in the Vienna General Hospital in the hope that he might be allowed to listen to the chests of patients. His incessant application of auscultation caused patients to complain. Hospital officials transferred Skoda to the mental patients' ward. But even these unfortunates wearied of Skoda's obsession for listening to their chests. He accepted a post as a physician to paupers, since they could not afford to complain about their doctors. Vindication came with Skoda's publication of a textbook, and he returned to the Vienna General Hospital in a higher capacity. Tapping and listening finally became an accepted technique of medicine with nineteenth-century physicians, who even stowed the stethoscope in their top hats.

The stethoscope carries two distinct sounds to the ear of the doctor. When the heart begins a contraction, the tricuspid and mitral valves (which lead from the right and left atria to their respective ventricles) slam shut. The

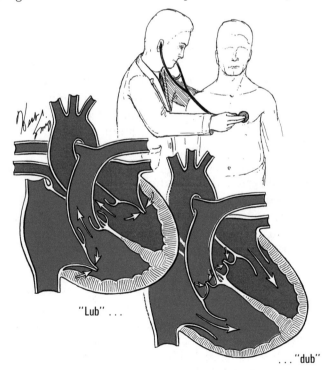

"Lub" . . .

. . . "dub"

Figure 16. The sounds a physician hears through the stethoscope are caused by the opening and closing of the various valves of the heart.

pulmonary and aortic valves (which are gates to the pulmonary artery and the aorta) open, and the leaves of these two valves vibrate from the pressure of the blood forcing them to expand. This tremor adds to the noise of the tricuspid and mitral valves closing, and a sound describable as a "lub" can be heard (Figure 16).

Just as the lub fades away, the pressure within the ventricles falls low enough for the aortic and pulmonary valves to swing shut, and a fraction of a second later the tricuspid and mitral valves open. This creates a vibrating noise which supplements the sound of the closing valves. To the ear at the end of the stethoscope comes a "dub." Then there is perceivable silence, since diastole ordinarily lasts longer than systole. The normal sequence heard is lub-dub, silence, lub-dub, silence.

Occasionally, vibrations of the ventricular cavity can be heard as it fills with blood pouring from the atria and a physician will hear a third sound. Through the stethoscope a doctor can hear if valves fail to close properly, or if some blood backs up into a ventricle instead of being pumped out. The normal heart rate of 70 beats per minute pumps little more than two and one-half fluid ounces per stroke which adds up to six quarts of output per minute. But when necessary, the heart can boost its performance to as much as thirty to thirty-five quarts per minute.

Pulse rate seems to bear some relation to the size of the species, varying from 1,000 beats per minute in a canary to about 25 beats per minute in an elephant. An infant's heart beats at about 120 beats per minute, while an adult's heart beats at 65 to 75 beats per minute. This rate in an adult adds up to approximately 100,000 beats per day or 2.5 billion in a lifetime. Pulse rate sharply increases with physical exertion, from a mild increase of 20 to 30 per minute upon walking, to more than twice as fast during sexual intercourse.

The cardiovascular system has computerlike ability to direct a heavier flow of blood to areas that require it, and detour around organs not needing it. This enhances circulatory efficiency. For example, gastric organs need an added amount of oxygenated blood during the digestion of food. But when no food is in the stomach, a series of shunts blocks off the flow of blood to these organs and the extra supply is then available to the legs and arms for physical work. This mechanism explains why athletes forego a meal just before engaging in competition.

The pump itself can contribute greatly to an increased supply of blood to needy tissues. The duration and even the intensity of cardiac systole (contraction) alters when the heart receives a demand for more oxygenated blood. In order for the blood to be pushed along faster, the time of diastole (relaxation) shortens. At rest, for example, systole lasts about one-third of a second and diastole about one-half of a second. During exercise the heart sustains the pressure stroke for perhaps one-fifth of a second and cuts its filling time to one-quarter of its normal time. The quantity of blood that is able to enter the heart drops and the output of oxygenated blood per stroke falls, although the total output per minute is, of course, much higher than normal.

Dr. Roger Bannister, the first person to run a mile in under four minutes, thinks that the enormous reduction in distance-running times is due to an increased blood oxygen efficiency that can result from training. In fact, Dr. Bannister predicts a 3.5-minute mile because of new methods to boost oxygen usage.

Let us consider the responses of the cardiovascular system to exercise. Visualize for a moment the safety man on a professional football team awaiting the punt at his goal line. His athletically trained heart may be beating about sixty times per minute at rest. However, in anticipation of the demands about to be placed upon his body, the player's sympathetic nervous system has already boosted his heart rate. In addition to the action of the nervous system, the adrenal glands have been stimulated to release adrenalin and noradrenalin, which initiate a series of reactions to prepare the player for "fright and flight." The player catches the ball and begins to run. Depending upon the degree of exertion and the rate of pursuit, his pulse rate may reach nearly 200 beats per minute and his cardiac output becomes as high as thirty-six quarts of blood per minute. This will almost certainly occur if he succeeds in running the full length of the field for a touchdown.

Ordinarily a healthy, trained athlete is unable to sustain exertion to the point that his heart muscle (myocardium) will suffer damage. Long before the myocardium reaches the danger point in terms of oxygen deficiency, other muscles in the body will suffer fatigue. It is indeed extraordinary to think that the heart must operate for seventy years without ever being permitted to rest or shut down for extensive repairs. It staggers the imagination to think of the wear and tear that the heart valves, those critically important parts of the cardiovascular machinery, must sustain in opening and shutting with considerable hydraulic pressure 2.5 billion times in a lifetime. The magnitude of these forces is apparent to a surgeon when replacing a defective heart valve with a *prosthetic device* consisting of a silicone ball in a steel cage. Some of these hard silicone balls become pitted, rutted and battered out of shape after only three or four years of being pounded by the blood. Because of this constant hammering, materials which are even stronger and more resilient than silicone are now being used (see Figure 104). Yet, in a normal, healthy heart, the delicate flesh of the valves stands up for seventy years or more.

Changes in cardiac output reflect biochemical and physiological adaptions of the muscle cells of the myocardium. There are two types of muscle cells in the body: striated and smooth. The skeletal or voluntary muscles that we call on to do physical work are made up of many individual striated cells, or fibrils (Figure 17). The muscle tissue of the heart is also composed of striated muscle cells, although it is not, of course, under voluntary control. Altogether, muscle accounts for approximately 40 to 50 percent of a person's weight. The individual muscle cell is a highly specialized structure whose function is to produce chemical energy that can be converted into mechanical work. Sustained contraction of muscles demands consumption of oxygen to burn fuels which provide the necessary energy.

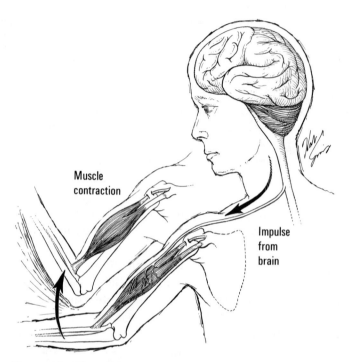

Muscle
contraction

Impulse
from
brain

Figure 17. The skeletal muscles of the body perform their mechanical function by contracting and relaxing in accordance with physical labor when electrical impulses are received from the brain through the nerves.

Both striated and smooth muscle cells contain myofibrils which are the basic structural units of the muscle (Figure 18). The substance surrounding the nucleus of the muscle cell is called the *sarcoplasm.* The sarcoplasm contains mitochondria and endoplasmic reticulum, similar to that of all cells. In the striated muscle, the myofibril contains multiple striations, or crossbands, while in the smooth muscle, no such striations are present.

The sequence of events that is thought to culminate in muscle contraction initiates with an electrical impulse from the nervous system which results in the electrical depolarization of the membrane of the cell (Figure 17).

The length of the muscle fiber prior to contraction is very important in determining the force developed during contraction. This is the basic principle behind the Frank Starling law of the heart. This law describes the functioning of the heart and states that the work done by the heart varies with the diastolic volume of the ventricle, which determines the length of the myocardial muscle fibers. Thus, when venous return to the heart is increased, there is an increased filling pressure of the heart, a rise in the diastolic volume

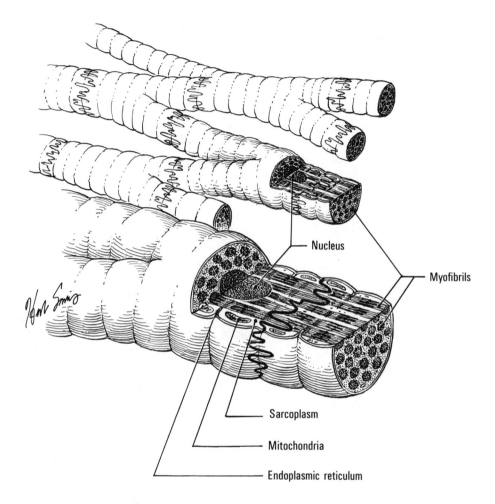

Figure 18. The structure of the striated muscle of the heart

and a greater stretching of the myocardial muscle fibers of the ventricle. This results in a higher stroke volume. When the heart is failing, the stroke volume produced by the left ventricle is decreased. In the failing heart, the contraction is inadequate for biological reasons that are still not clearly understood. One possibility is that there is a dysfunction between the coupling of the chemical energy and the mechanical work to be done by the heart. When the heart fails, there is insufficient mechanical energy to adequately pump blood to meet the needs of the body's tissues. The drug *digitalis* tends to increase the contractile force of the failing heart.

When the body is subjected to physical exertion, there is an increase in the amount of oxygen used by the tissues. In order to provide enough oxygen, the body responds by increasing the output of the heart, largely through a faster pulse rate, a more rapid rate of respiration, and by an increase in the amount of oxygen extracted from the bloodstream by organs and tissues. Cardiac output also is increased through a decrease in the resistance to blood flow near the extremities of the cardiovascular system. In another of nature's ingenious engineering triumphs, a sensing mechanism reduces resistance to the flow of blood by widening the blood vessels which supply the working muscle tissue.

If an individual is in good physical health, his oxygen will be supplied at a slower pulse rate than it is in a person in poor condition. While both individuals can reach the same maximal pulse rate for their age, the subject in good condition is able to achieve a higher level of work due to the greater amount of oxygen that can be carried to and extracted by the tissues. This maximum oxygen uptake reached by an individual during exercise is sometimes referred to as the "aerobic capacity." This capacity declines as people get older and can be decreased further by cardiovascular disease or other forms of illness.

The conversion of chemical energy into mechanical work by muscle can be achieved only by shortening of the fibers or by an increase in their tension. A number of years ago, the great physiologist A. V. Hill described the fundamental relationship between these two parameters, which in simple terms states that the rate of shortening of the muscle fiber varies inversely with the degree of tension achieved. Thus, if tension is great, as when lifting a heavy object, the shortening of the muscle will occur at a relatively slow velocity. On the other hand, if a light object is to be raised, requiring only a small degree of tension, the rate of shortening will be much faster. Changes in the contractile state of the heart muscle may be altered by varying the resting length of the muscle fiber or by changing the contractility of the fiber. Practical ways to accomplish this are by giving drugs such as noradrenalin or digitalis, both of which increase the force and velocity of contraction that the heart can achieve.

Maintenance of the normal *contractility of the heart* depends upon innervation by sympathetic nerve endings which release noradrenalin. This sympathetic control tends to speed up the heart, increase the rate at which the muscle fibers contract and augment the pace at which the left ventricle ejects the blood.

During exercise, there is an increase in ventricular filling pressure due to an increase in the venous return to the heart. At the same time, the sympathetic nerve fibers and the circulating adrenalin and noradrenalin speed up the rate of the heart and increase venous return to the heart. The sympathetic nerve fibers and the circulating adrenalin and noradrenalin also increase the contractility of the myocardium. All of these forces tend to increase the diastolic volume and the length of the heart fibers, greatly augmenting cardiac output.

These changes occur to a lesser degree or not at all in the failing heart. In heart failure, the pumping action of the heart is inadequate to meet the metabolic demands of the tissues. It is important to emphasize that the exact biochemical basis for ordinary heart failure is not known. There appears to be a decrease in the amount of noradrenalin stored and released. Whatever the cause, there is simply a diminished output of the heart in relation to tissue demands. The most common causes of this type of heart failure are *atherosclerotic coronary artery disease, hypertension* and *valvular disease.* Energy production by the heart appears to be normal, but its capacity to produce useful mechanical work is impaired. Heart failure may also be caused by *pulmonary embolism,* by an infection of the heart valves known as bacterial endocarditis, by severe systemic infection or by other heart abnormalities.

Clinical manifestations of heart failure include fluid accumulation in the peripheral tissues (particularly the legs), the liver and the lungs. Pulmonary congestion and eventually a highly dangerous condition known as *pulmonary edema* may result. The old term "dropsy" was used to describe congestive heart failure. This condition is characterized by a shortness of breath upon exertion, and an abnormal degree of fatigue and weakness. It is a rarity when heart failure is a "high output" rather than a "low output" type. High output heart failure may result from thiamine deficiency in beriberi, hyperthyroidism, severe anemia and arterio-venous fistula.

Digitalis and *noradrenalin* administered to a patient may improve the contractility of a failing heart. Drugs, such as barbiturates, and conditions such as *myocardial infarction,* severe *hypoxia* or *acidosis* may depress the contractility of the myocardium. When heart failure cannot be corrected by medical measures, surgical treatment in the form of a cardiac assist device may sometimes be employed.

Muscular efforts are one type of request for additional work by the heart, but there are others. The poetry of Shakespeare and the most contemporary of folk-rock ballad writers point to the heart as a tail wagged at varying speeds by one's emotions. In everyday life we become aware of subtle changes in heartbeat caused by some sensory or intellectual perception. The sight of an attractive member of the opposite sex can turn the heartbeat from a stately cadence to a quick step. This is caused by a signal from the brain which receives information from the eye and combines it with certain stored impressions to produce an increased heartbeat. Two separate nerve lines link heart and brain, the sympathetic, or accelerator, nerves which liberate noradrenalin, and the vagus system which tends to slow the heart (Figure 19).

The vagus system is a major influence in depressing the frequency of impulses from the "pacemaker" sinoatrial node of the heart. Sometimes surgical repair of the heart cuts the vagal connection and, inevitably, the patient's heartbeat, even while at rest, exceeds the accepted norm. The accelerator system reaches beyond the heart's pacemaker nodes and can be traced into the heart muscle itself. In extreme surgery, such as a heart transplant, where accelerator and vagus lines into the heart have been severed, the nervous system can no longer affect the heart rate. But the heart still retains a regular rhythm through its own pacemaker, the sinoatrial node and its relay to the atrioventricular node. While the heart is capable of generating its own rhythm, in a healthy body its tempo and electrical activity are, in fact, modulated by impulses from the brain.

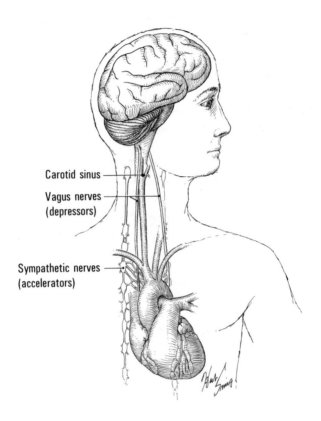

Carotid sinus

Vagus nerves
(depressors)

Sympathetic nerves
(accelerators)

Figure 19. The heart rate is controlled by electrical impulses
from the brain through the vagus and sympathetic nerves.

A major advance in the study of the physiology of the heart was the discovery that the electrical discharge from the two cardiac nodes provides an excellent means to measure heart action by means of electrocardiography.

As early as 1856, two German scientists reported that the heartbeat of a frog was accompanied by an electrical impulse. Researchers experimented with measurement of this current in animals. But not until a London physiologist, Augustus Waller, learned how to record this electrical impulse without opening the patient's chest, was it deemed possible to work with humans. Waller gave the technology a name, electrocardiography, but not even he thought it more than just an interesting toy. The problem was that Waller's machine lacked stability and the capacity to precisely follow the

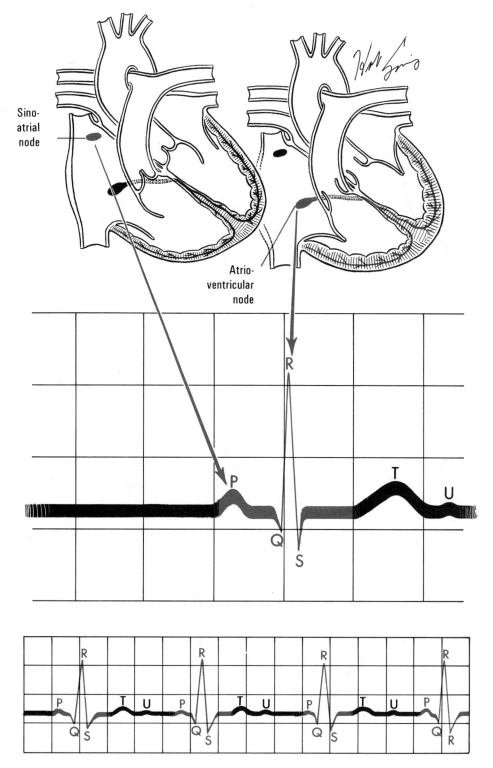

Sino-
atrial
node

Atrio-
ventricular
node

Figure 20. The electrocardiogram records the electrical activity of the conduction system of the heart.

rapid changes in the minute variations of current associated with the heartbeat.

The need for an instrument adequate to register electrical current in the heart attracted the attention of a physiology professor named Willem Einthoven at the University of Utrecht. Starting in 1893, he worked for seven years on the problem of designing a more satisfactory machine. The result was what Einthoven called the "string galvanometer." The electrical current flowed from electrodes in the body's surface through a quartz thread. The thread was suspended in the force field of an electromagnet which vibrated as the current flowing through it interacted with the force field. An optical system focused the shadow cast by the quartz thread upon a light-sensitive surface which recorded its deflections. This Rube Goldberg-like machine weighed six hundred pounds and needed five technicians to operate properly. But the *electrocardiograms* provided such superior records of heart activity that Einthoven subsequently earned a Nobel Prize.

Invention of vacuum tubes did away with the cumbersome string galvanometer machines. The weight of a modern electrocardiography unit amounts to perhaps thirty pounds, with only one person needed to run it. In operating rooms and intensive care units, cathode ray oscilloscope versions monitor cardiac performance, and electrical impulses of the heart send beams of electrons dancing across a screen for an immediately visible record of heart function. To chart the passage of the electrical impulse, a technician places electrodes, or receivers of current, on the chest, arms and legs. The machine then records the passage of electrical energy from the heart on a graph. The amount of voltage of these impulses is only a matter of millivolts, yet these tiny impulses are enough to excite heart muscle. On a normal *electrocardiogram* each vertical line represents one-fifth of a second in time and the horizontal lines indicate one-half of a millivolt (Figure 20).

The measurement begins with the P wave, which indicates the discharge of electrical energy by the sinoatrial (SA) node, which swiftly fans out over the right and left atria. This electrical phenomenon is called depolarization. The P wave thus reflects the activation of the atria. The QRS segment follows the subsequent depolarization of the atrioventricular (AV) node, and reflects the electrical current's journey through the conduction system of the heart and into the muscular walls of the right and left ventricles. Portions of the conduction pathway beyond the AV node are called the bundle of His; the left and right bundle branches supply the left and right ventricles. Measurement of the interval between the P wave and the R wave indicates the length of time between the discharges of the SA node and the AV node. The first downward (negative) deflection of the QRS complex is designated as the Q wave, the initial upward (positive) deflection the R wave and the second negative deflection is the S wave. The T wave indicates how long it takes for the recharging (repolarization) of the ventricles. From the distance between the Q and T waves, the physician observes the duration of excitation, ventricular contraction, and repolarization or recovery of the heart.

By recording an electrocardiogram over a period of time, a physician can see irregularities in the rhythm of a heart. Sometimes a patient will be asked to run in place so that his cardiogram can show the effect of exercise upon the heart. But whether the body is at rest or in motion the heart's rhythm should accelerate and decelerate smoothly. Abnormal rhythms and rates on the

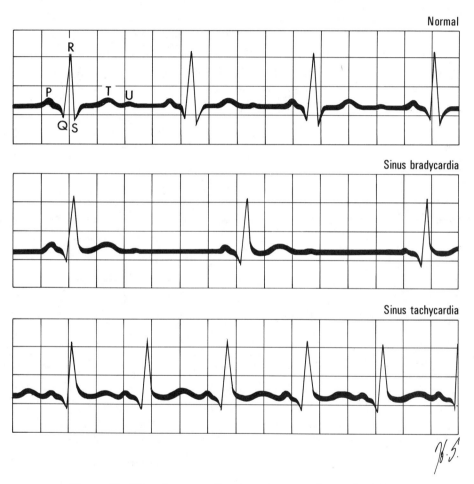

Figure 21. The electrocardiogram shows a slower heartbeat during sinus bradycardia and a faster rhythm during sinus tachycardia.

electrocardiogram are indications of malfunction. Occasionally, an individual will have an abnormal rhythm that actually works fine for him. If the physician has kept a series of electrocardiograms on this patient over a period of years, the seemingly aberrant heart action will not be disturbing—for this particular heart, the action is normal. On the other hand, a slight variation in the cardiogram of an individual whose previous medical history showed a perfectly normal graph may indicate serious trouble. For this reason, we urge regular electrocardiography as part of everyone's annual physical examination, and exercise cardiograms for adults who are about to undertake a new program of physical exercise.

An abnormality of cardiac rate, or rhythm, is called an *arrhythmia*. The commonest is a slowing of the heart to less than fifty beats per minute, usually due to an excess of vagal inhibition at the SA node. This condition is called sinus bradycardia (Figure 21). Athletes may have a slow pulse and sinus bradycardia as their normal rhythm. Emotional excitement may produce the opposite effect, sinus tachycardia, in which the pulse rate is greater than 100 beats per minute. A decrease in vagal tone or an increase in the sympathetic or accelerator nerve activity usually produces this rhythm.

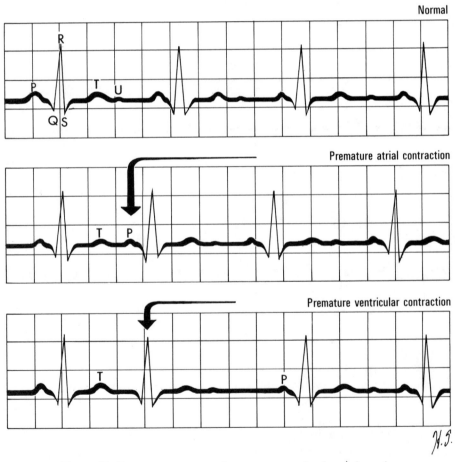

Figure 22. Premature contractions can occur in the atria or in the ventricles.

Hyperthyroidism, congestive heart failure and fever are all causes of sinus tachycardia.

An arrhythmia that arises outside the normal conduction pathway of the heart is called an ectopic focus. Such a focus generally represents an area of irritability within the myocardium. An ectopic stimulus arising from the muscle of the atria can produce premature atrial contractions, while one coming from the ventricles can cause premature ventricular contractions (Figure 22). In order to induce a premature beat, the irritable focus of electrical activity must stimulate the heart muscle at a point in the cardiac cycle when it is susceptible to activation. The heart is vulnerable to reactivation at about the time of the T wave. The particular type of arrhythmia induced depends upon the precise timing in the cardiac cycle when the irritable focus discharges, as well as its location within the heart. Premature atrial or ventricular beats may occur with almost any type of heart disease, particularly coronary artery disease. Excessive fatigue, smoking, coffee and other stimulants, emotional stress, febrile illness and various metabolic and electrolyte disturbances can precipitate premature beats in the normal heart. Premature ventricular beats frequently occur during heart catheterization, after heart surgery or during a heart attack.

Premature contractions may be perceived by the patient as a skipped beat. In the absence of underlying heart disease, premature atrial and occasional premature ventricular beats may be effectively treated by rest, sedatives and withdrawal of stimulants. If there is underlying heart disease or if premature ventricular contractions become too frequent, the use of an antiarrhythmic drug may be indicated. For an individual patient, the choice of drug depends upon the type of arrhythmia and the cardiac and clinical status.

In addition to premature contractions, other frequently encountered atrial arrhythmias include paroxysmal atrial tachycardia, atrial flutter and atrial fibrillation (Figure 23). In paroxysmal atrial tachycardia, an irritable atrial focus takes over from the normal pacemaker, namely, the SA node, and the pulse rate usually accelerates to about 180 beats per minute. Premature atrial beats usually precede arrhythmia. This cardiac irregularity may occur periodically in otherwise normal individuals or it may be caused by coronary or rheumatic heart disease or by an overactive thyroid. Fatigue, stimulants and emotional stress may bring on attacks. A patient may learn to terminate an attack by gagging or by external massage of the carotid sinus in the neck, procedures which increase vagal tone.

In atrial flutter, which has a similar origin to paroxysmal atrial tachycardia, the atrial rate is 250 to 400 beats per minute. The ventricle is unable to respond this rapidly so that a form of heart block occurs at the AV node and the ventricular rate is usually 150 to 200 beats per minute and is regular. This means that not every atrial contraction on the electrocardiogram is followed by a QRS complex, due to the absence of a 1:1 ventricular response. The P waves are abnormal in atrial flutter, having a "saw-toothed" configuration. Atrial flutter is usually treated with antiarrhythmic drugs.

In contrast to atrial flutter, which is not common, atrial fibrillation is very frequently encountered in patients with heart disease, either of coronary

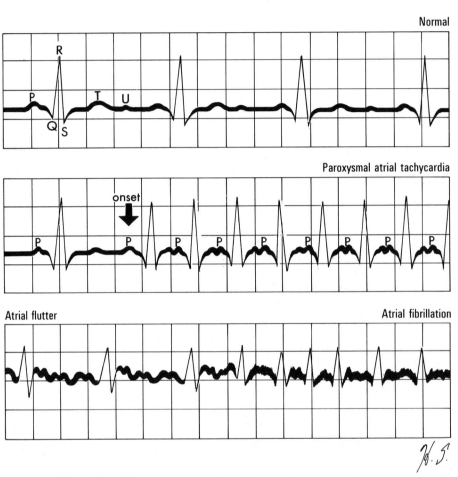

Figure 23. When paroxysmal atrial tachycardia occurs, the heartbeat increases to about 180 beats per minute. When atrial flutter occurs, the rate increases to over 250 per minute. In atrial fibrillation, the atria contract in an irregular and ineffective way.

or rheumatic *etiology*. In this condition an abnormal atrial focus discharges at a rate greater than 350 beats per minute. As a consequence, the atria do not contract in an effective or organized way. The AV node and the ventricles respond irregularly. Clinical manifestations depend upon the rate of the ventricular response. If this rate is so rapid that the ventricles do not have adequate time to fill, heart failure may ensue. A digitalis preparation is usually given to slow or control the ventricular rate. Patients live many years and carry on their daily functions perfectly well with a properly slowed atrial fibrillation. The pulse is still irregular, however, even when the arrhythmia is well regulated. In some instances after digitalization, it may be possible to convert a patient from atrial fibrillation to a sinus rhythm by giving the drug quinidine or by electric countershock. A potentially serious complication of atrial fibrillation is that a blood clot, or thrombus, can form within the atria and subsequently dislodge to enter the arterial circulation. A serious stroke, or cerebrovascular accident, may occur if the dislodged thrombus, now called an embolus, is carried to the brain. The electrocardiogram in atrial filbrillation shows normal, but irregularly spaced, QRS complexes and absent P waves.

The arrhythmias, ventricular tachycardia, ventricular fibrillation and ventricular standstill are of a very serious nature (Figure 24). Ventricular tachycardia arises from an irritable focus in the myocardium and usually indicates underlying heart disease, especially atherosclerotic coronary disease. This irregularity resembles a series of premature ventricular beats and produces a rate of 140 to 220 beats per minute. Ventricular filling falls off and heart failure may follow. The pulse may be absent at the wrist and, if untreated, the patient may go into cardiogenic shock. Intravenous administration of medication or administration of electric countershock is required and may save the patient's life.

In ventricular fibrillation, the ventricular muscles cannot maintain a coordinated contraction in response to an exceedingly rapid irritable focus. The muscle goes into a kind of rapid twitching and consequently does not effectively pump blood. In ventricular standstill, there is no impulse to stimulate the ventricle, and the muscle, in a sense, stands still. Ventricular fibrillation and ventricular standstill produce the condition called cardiac arrest in which there is no detectable heartbeat, pulse or blood pressure. Breathing usually stops; the patient loses consciousness and will suffer irreversible brain damage unless resuscitation or correction of the arrhythmia is carried out within four to six minutes. In a coronary care unit, the occurrence of a cardiac arrest triggers a number of emergency measures aimed at correcting the condition: The arrhythmia must be corrected by electric countershock; respiration and the blood pressure must be supported; and acidosis must be reversed. If the arrest occurs outside an area where a defibrillator is available to produce the countershock, cardiopulmonary resuscitation must be instituted. As illustrated in Figure 25, this procedure involves breathing air into the victim's lungs and applying external cardiac massage to pump the blood out of the heart. Courses in cardiopulmonary resuscitation (CPR) are available to the layman through the American Heart Association and the Red Cross. Being able to carry out CPR may enable you to actually save someone's life.

There is another group of heart irregularities known collectively as heart

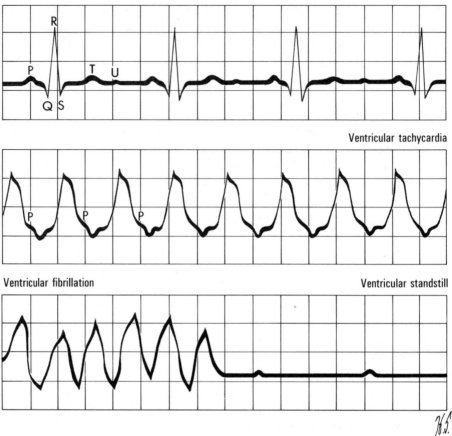

Figure 24. In ventricular tachycardia, the heartbeat increases to 140 to 220 beats per minute. In ventricular fibrillation, the heart muscle goes into uncoordinated spasmodic contractions and does not effectively pump blood. In ventricular standstill there is no impulse to stimulate the ventricle.

block (Figure 26). The cause of this type of arrhythmia is an interference with the normal conduction system of the heart as the impulses pass through the AV node. The heart block may be first degree, second degree or third degree. In first degree heart block, there is a 1:1 response of atrial and ventricular contractions, but a slowing of conduction through the AV node to produce an increased P-R interval on the electrocardiogram. In second degree block, some of the impulses do not pass through the AV node and the atrial to ventricular response is not 1:1 but instead 2:1, 3:1, etc. In second degree heart block, some of the P waves are not followed by a QRS complex. In third degree heart block, there is no conduction through the AV node. A slow ventricular rate occurs due to the fact that a pacemaker within the ventricle itself takes over. In complete heart block, there is no relationship between the atrial beats or P waves and the QRS complexes.

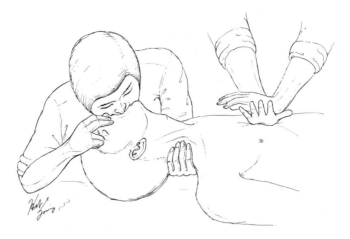

Figure 25. Cardiopulmonary resuscitation involves breathing air into the victim's lungs and applying external heart massage.

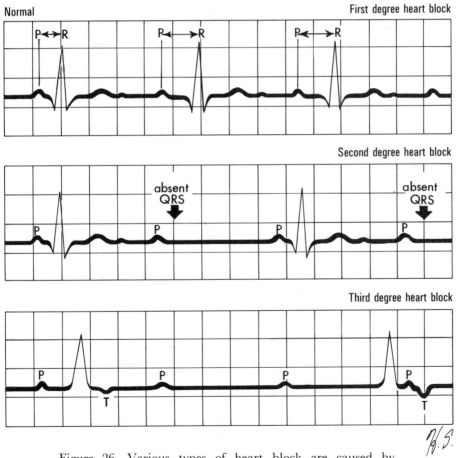

Figure 26. Various types of heart block are caused by interference with the normal conduction system of the heart.

If the heart rate slows to the point that the ventricle cannot pump an adequate amount of blood to support the requirements of the body, particularly the brain, heart failure and unconsciousness rapidly occur. The patient with complete heart block may develop cardiac arrest or ventricular fibrillation, a potentially lethal situation. Loss of consciousness in association with third degree heart block is called Stokes-Adams attack. Second degree or third degree heart block may require treatment if the ventricular rate is not adequate. The drug isoproterenol or ephedrine may be given to increase the heart rate in complete heart block. In some instances it is necessary to insert a pacemaker to control complete heart block. This use of pacemakers is discussed in Chapter 15.

In concluding this chapter, it may be useful to review some of the awesome statistics concerning the heart and place them in another frame of reference. For example, the 60,000 miles of blood vessels in each adult equals a trip of nearly two and one-half times around the world, or a quarter of the distance from the earth to the moon. A single heart that pumps six quarts of blood per minute (360 quarts per hour) by the end of seventy years would have moved over 220 million quarts, a number exceeding the population of the United States. It's a pretty remarkable piece of machinery.

5

THE

VASCULAR SYSTEM

THE heart, as we have said, is the center of the cardiovascular system. The body's requirement for oxygen and food is met by a network of blood vessels known as the vascular, or circulatory, system. As William Harvey discovered, this system is a continous network, connected with the heart, which serves as a pump. The blood vessels comprising the vascular system consist of arteries, arterioles, capillaries, venules and veins (Figure 27). It is important to keep in mind that this is a closed system of vessels with a lining called the endothelium. The blood vessels transport the blood from the heart to the tissues of the body and back again; they may be compared to a network of highways, roads and channels through which cargo (the blood) is continously pumped by the heart to supply the needs of the body.

Blood, primed with oxygen, leaves the heart on its journey via a large artery called the aorta. From the aorta, the blood travels through smaller arteries and then arterioles to connect with a network of vessels known as capillaries. As blood moves from the heart to the capillary bed, the arteries become progressively smaller and more numerous. Their total cross-sectional area increases so that the rate of flow of the blood decreases as it gets farther away from the heart.

The arteries themselves range from a great superhighway, the aorta, with its one-inch diameter, down to the minute arterioles, whose width is

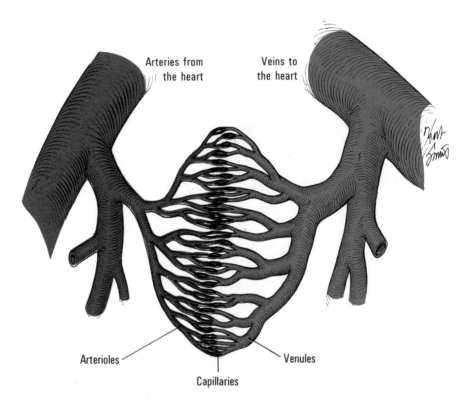

Arteries from
the heart

Veins to
the heart

Arterioles

Venules

Capillaries

Figure 27. From the heart, oxygenated blood passes from the arteries through smaller branches called arterioles into the capillaries, where food and oxygen are supplied to the cells of the body and waste products are removed. After passing through the capillaries, the blood enters the small venules, which connect to the veins to return the blood to the heart.

only about 0.02 of an inch. The capillaries, the final passageways for the blood, are smaller than a single red cell which must bend and squirm to pass through. Along these avenues of transport lie many of the potential dangers of life.

An artery's wall may be divided into three layers, or sections: the *intima,* the *media* and the *adventitia* (Figure 28). The innermost layer of the artery is called the intima. At birth it is only one cell thick and consists of the endothelium, the lining which is in direct contact with the blood. Hardening of the arteries, referred to as arteriosclerosis or atherosclerosis, probably begins with damage to the endothelial lining, permitting fatty substances and other toxic agents into the intima (see Chapter 8). A thin structure, the internal elastic membrane, separates the intima from a muscular coat called the media of the artery's wall.

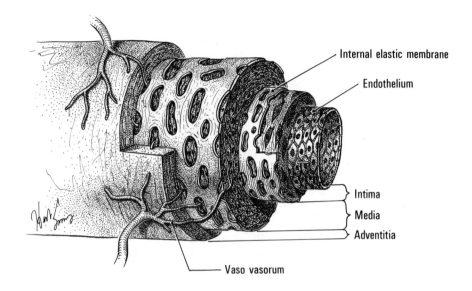

Figure 28. The different types of cellular components of the three layers that constitute the structure of an artery

Large arteries nearer the heart are subjected to the strong pulsations generated as this organ contracts. They are protected from the pounding action of the heart by virtue of being able to recoil, a property that depends on the media being relatively rich in elastic tissue (*elastin*). The pulsations decrease in intensity further from the heart so that the smaller the artery, the greater its ratio of muscle tissue to elastin. The smooth muscle cell of the artery's media may play a key role in the development of arteriosclerosis, which is the disease underlying most heart attacks and strokes. The outermost layer of the artery's wall, the adventitia, is rich in connective tissue, nerve fibers and a special group of blood vessels called the *vasa vasorum,* which supply the artery itself. The vasa vasorum is a network of small vessels which provide oxygen-filled blood for the walls of medium-sized and large arteries and veins.

When the wall becomes thickened, as in the vessel affected by arteriosclerosis, the diffusion of oxygen to the center of the media may not be sufficient, leading to cell death and further damage to the artery.

The state of contraction of muscular arteries is regulated by sympathetic nerve fibers which are abundant in the adventitia. Arterioles, which are the smallest of arteries, are of particular importance in determining the level of the arterial blood pressure. Relaxation, or dilation, of the arterioles decreases the resistance to blood flow and lowers the blood pressure. Vasoconstrictor nerve fibers, part of the sympathetic nervous system, release adrenalin and noradrenalin to regulate the contractile tone of the arterioles. An excessive degree of arteriole contraction is thought to be one of the important causes of high blood pressure, or hypertension, in which there is a persistent elevation of the arterial blood pressure.

The smallest arterioles merge with capillaries of the same size, the distinction between these two types of vessels being the total absence of a muscular layer in the capillary. Thus, the capillary consists of only a layer of endothelium surrounded by connective tissue.

Capillaries empty into venules which, in turn, form veins. The vein has a larger *lumen* and a thinner wall with relatively less muscle and elastic tissue than an artery of the same size. The relatively larger lumen accounts for the slower flow of blood and lower pressure in the venous system.

If one were to tour the body via the vascular system, the journey would begin with a departure from the left ventricle through the aortic valve. Just beyond the aortic valve are the coronary arteries and their network of branches which supply blood to the heart itself (Figure 29). These arteries girdle the heart like a crown, hence the name coronary. They account for five

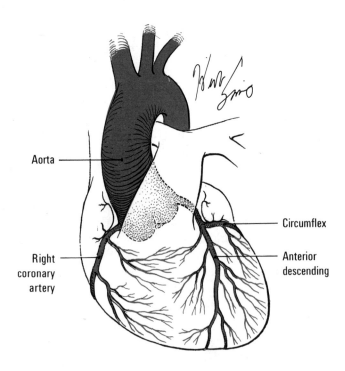

Figure 29. The coronary arteries, which arise from the aorta just above the aortic valve, provide blood for the various tissues of the heart.

percent of the total blood flow, although their diameter at most equals that of a thick piece of twine or a soda straw. A healthy heart, particularly one developed through a regular program of exercise, shows an extensive field of blood vessels flowing from the coronary arteries.

Immediately beyond the exit of the coronary artery comes the *aortic arch,* which forms two major channels leading from the heart, one to the lower part of the body and the other to the upper part, especially the brain (Figure 30).

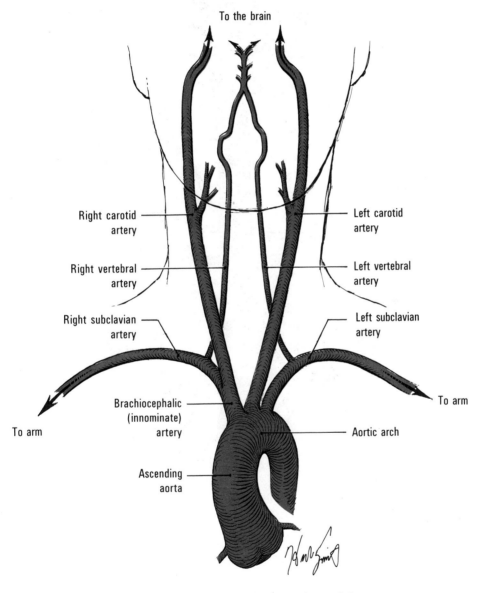

Figure 30. Three major arteries—the innominate, left common carotid and left subclavian—arise from the aortic arch to supply the head and arms with blood.

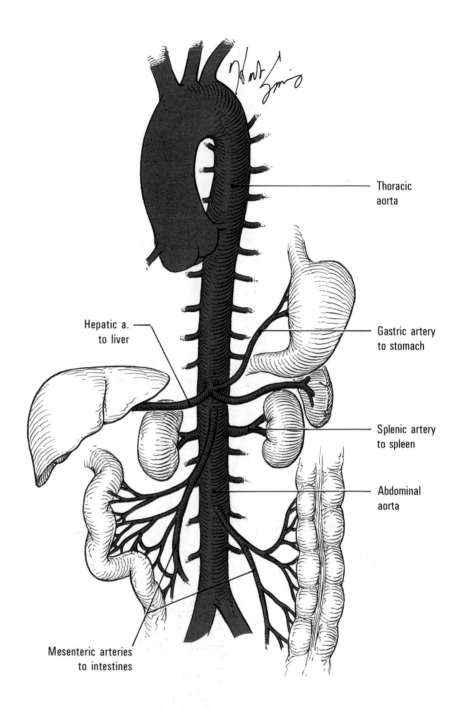

Thoracic
aorta

Hepatic a.
to liver

Gastric artery
to stomach

Splenic artery
to spleen

Abdominal
aorta

Mesenteric arteries
to intestines

Figure 31. Branches arise from the aorta in the chest and
abdomen to supply blood to the body wall and major organs.

The upper channel is formed by three major vessels that arise from the
ascending aorta; they are the *innominate*, the left common *carotid* and the left
subclavian arteries. The innominate divides into the right subclavian and the

right common carotid arteries. The subclavian arteries feed the left and right chest, shoulders and arms through their branches. The left and right common carotid arteries carry blood to the neck and head.

Arteriosclerotic disease of the carotid arteries may lead to cerebrovascular disease and stroke. Some additional blood flows to the head through the vertebral arteries which branch from the subclavians. Inside the skull, a vast network of arteries feed the cells of the brain. The main arteries supplying the brain form a circle at its base called the *circle of Willis*. This circle of arteries serves to provide all parts of the brain with relatively equal amounts of blood.

The arterial route to the lower half of the body starts at the downturn of the aortic arch. As the aorta passes through the diaphragm, it becomes the abdominal aorta (Figure 31). A series of crossroads fan out to supply organs and tissue along the way. Each major organ has its own route; gastric arteries supply the stomach, hepatic arteries go to the liver, and renal arteries feed the kidneys. The kidney has a special relationship to the cardiovascular system, filtering approximately 150 quarts of blood every twenty-four hours to remove wastes from the system.

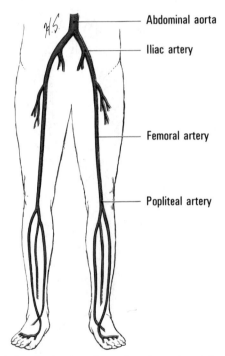

Figure 32. The abdominal aorta branches into the right and left iliac arteries to supply blood to the thighs and legs.

Below the stomach, the abdominal aorta branches into the right and left *iliac arteries* to supply the thighs and legs (Figure 32). Further subdivisions occur as the system extends to the lower legs, the feet and finally the toes.

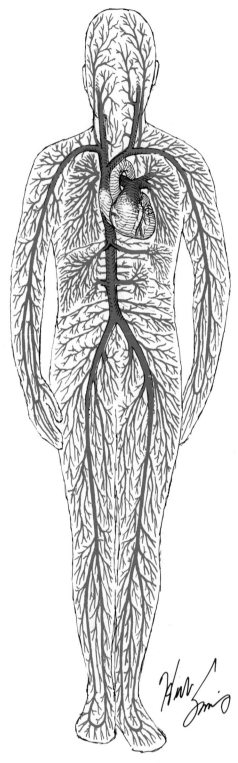

Figure 33. The venous system returns blood from the various tissues of the body to the heart.

Sideroads from the arteries fan out into a maze of smaller and smaller vessels, until the arterioles and capillaries are reached. The capillaries pass through the spaces between cells where the delicate transfer of food and oxygen in exchange for waste occurs.

In the spleen and bone marrow, the capillaries may empty into tissue spaces. However, this is an exception, and the endothelium of the capillary is usually continuous with that of venules and veins, which convey the blood back to the heart and lungs. Because the oxygen tension is low in peripheral tissues, venous blood appears bluish (Figure 33).

During the early part of the trip, a strong pressure was generated by the contractions of the heart. The force is dissipated by the time blood reaches the veins and the outward rush of blood from the heart gives small impetus to the return flow. The push for the trip through the venous system comes from the normal use of leg, arm, back and stomach muscles that squeeze the veins

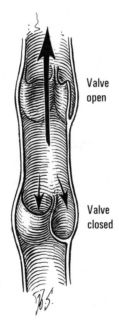

Valve
open

Valve
closed

Figure 34. One-way valves in the veins prevent blood from flowing backward.

whenever a human walks, writes, lifts or even rolls over in his sleep. Because of the relative scarcity of muscle and elastic tissue in its wall, a vein is more easily compressed by adjacent muscles and bones than is the artery. This phenomenon is important in promoting the return of blood to the heart from the limbs, which must flow against the force of gravity, particularly when a person is standing. In addition to the compressibility of the vein, the other significant factor in the antigravity flow is the presence of valves in veins. These one-way valves prevent blood from oozing backward (Figure 34). If the valves of the leg veins become impaired and allow a backward flow to occur, the blood tends to pool in the limb, distending the veins and resulting in varicosities. The presence of varicose veins is not however, to be confused with arterial disease; these varicosities are unrelated to arteriosclerosis.

Normally, blood pressure which is measured in millimeters of mercury during the contraction of the heart (systole), reaches around 110-140 in a young adult. During the relaxed phase of the heart (diastole), pressure falls to

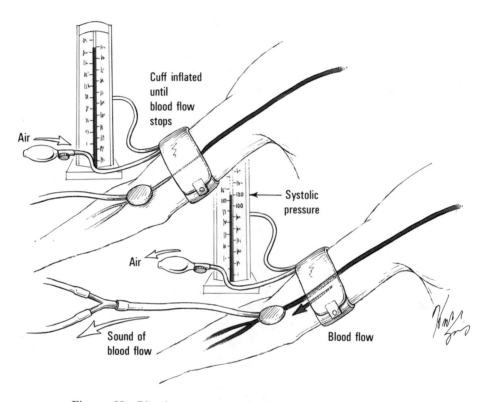

Figure 35. Blood pressure is determined by listening for certain changes in the sound of blood flowing through artery as the pressure in the pneumatic cuff, which has been raised sufficiently to cut off arterial blood flow, is gradually decreased.

70-90. An English parson, the Reverend Stephen Hales, performed the first experiment designed to measure blood pressure. He trussed up a horse, then inserted a glass tube, a primitive device for measuring fluid pressure, in an artery on the horse's neck. The column of blood rose to seven and one-half feet and Hales established that as normal blood pressure in a horse.

Inconvenient for the physician, to say nothing of the patient, (Reverend Hales sacrificed seven animals in the course of his experiments), the technique obviously required improvement. In 1828, Jean Marie Poiseuille succeeded in reducing the size of the tube by designing a U-shaped device filled with mercury, which is 13.6 times as heavy as water. Blood pressure could now be measured by the millimeter height of a column of mercury. Poiseuille also corrected one of Reverend Hale's errors. The clergyman concluded that blood pressure drops as arterial distance from the heart increases. Poiseuille constructed cannulas or tubes small enough to insert into the smaller arteries and discovered that arterial pressure maintains a steady level throughout the system.

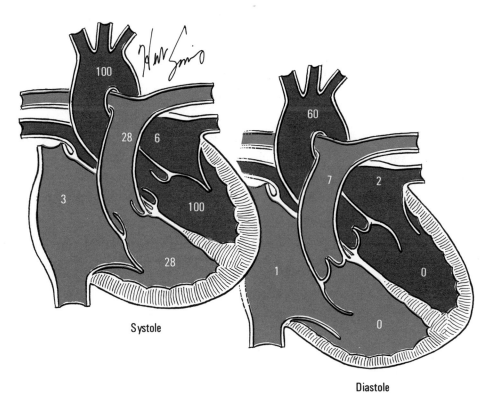

Figure 36. Normal pressures (in millimeters of mercury) in the various chambers of the heart

Still the need to open an artery in order to measure blood pressure restricted this valuable information to use in the experimental laboratory and had no useful clinical application. Practitioners in the second half of the nineteenth century began probing for methods that would enable them to determine how much pressure was required to obliterate the pulse beat in the radial artery at the wrist. In 1863, Étienne Jules Marey and Koming Dudgeon of France, both built simple machines to record the frequency of pulse beats. A young British doctor, Frederick Akhbar Mahomed, modified

Marey's device. He measured the amount of thumbscrew pressure required to stop blood flow in the wrist. Some individuals whose pulse beat required excessive pressure were found to have *nephritis,* a kidney disease which produces an acute elevation of blood pressure. But Dr. Mahomed's chief contribution was in showing a way to measure blood pressure without entering a blood vessel.

Others continued to improve machines to gauge the force of blood pumped by the heart. The device currently used is called a sphygmomanometer—the initial seven letters come from the Greek word for throb. There are several forms, each named for the individual who devised it. One such device was designed in 1896 by the Italian physician Dr. Sciopioni Riva-Rocci. An inflatable *pneumatic cuff* around the arm is used to constrict the brachial artery (Figure 35). Squeezing an inflatable bulb, the examiner raises the pressure in the cuff and listens with the stethoscope on the arm just below the cuff. While the pressure in the cuff is lower than in the artery, some blood can flow through the vessel, and the sound of its turbulent passage can be heard through the stethoscope. Excessive pumping on the inflatable bulb tightens the cuff enough to shut off the circulation and the sound stops. Gradually, air is released from the cuff. As cuff pressure drops below the level of the arterial blood pressure, the examiner hears the distinct noise of renewed blood flow. The cycle of sounds associated with the measurement of systolic and diastolic blood pressure was first described by Nicolai Korotoff and bears his name. These sounds are thought to be caused by a sudden distention of the arterial walls from a previous state of collapse, as the pressure in the pneumatic cuff is lessened. The height of the column of mercury when the pressure in the artery surpasses that of the inflated cuff is the systolic pressure. The diastolic pressure is registered as more air drains from the cuff and a change in the character of the sounds is heard. Some observers record the pressure level at which these sounds disappear altogether.

Although an electrical impulse originating in the heart's pacemaker activates the heart's cycle of contraction and relaxation, the dynamics of the cardiovascular system depend upon hydraulic pressure (Figure 36). During diastole, the period of relaxation of heart muscle and filling of the ventricles, blood pressure in the aorta is as much as fifteen times that of the ventricle. It takes one-tenth of a second for the cardiac muscle to contract enough to surpass the aortic pressure and force open the aortic valve.

While the blood pours from the heart in spasmodic spurts, it travels through the arterial system at a more even pressure, similar to water coursing through a hose. The intermittent flow of blood from the heart turns into a steadier stream because of the elastic muscle fibers that gird the arteries. As each beat of the heart pushes a greater volume of blood into the aorta, its fibers relax, increasing the cubic volume in which the blood circulates and lowering the pressure (Figure 37). During diastole, as the heart muscle relaxes, blood flow slackens, and the aorta shrinks its size to maintain pressure. Other large arteries possess the same flexible quality to keep pressure even. When a person becomes active and the tissues need more oxygen and other nutriments, the arterioles relax and resistance drops to help speed along the supplies through the capillaries.

More than three hundred years ago, William Harvey proclaimed an appropriate conclusion for this chapter: " ... by good leave of the learned

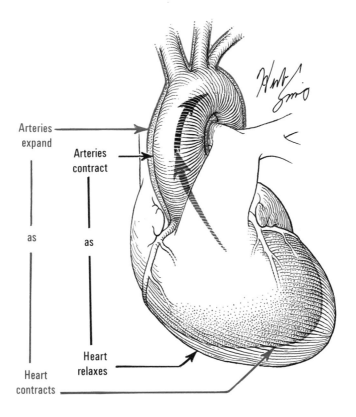

Figure 37. The arteries expand and contract to aid the heart
in pumping blood throughout the body.

and with due respect to the ancients, that the heart, as the beginning, author, source and organ of everything in the body and the first cause of life, should be held to include the veins and all the arteries and also the contained blood, just as the brain including all its nerves and sensory organs and spinal marrow is the one adequate organ of sensation as the phrase is. If by the word 'heart' however, only the body of the heart be meant with its ventricles and auricles I do not believe that it is the manufacturer of the blood nor that blood possesses vigor, faculty."

In fact, Harvey understated the case. With the limited knowledge of his time, he was unaware of roles played by the kidneys, liver and lungs in "the first cause of life," and he wasn't cognizant of the cardiovascular system's role in causing strokes. But he pointed the way to understanding why we suffer cardiovascular disease and what can be done to protect our bodies and help us recover in the event of a heart attack.

6

DEVELOPMENTS IN
CARDIOVASCULAR
SURGERY

*F*EW medical specialties have shown the phenomenal progress that cardiovascular surgery has made during the past several decades. A number of factors are responsible for this substantial advancement and among the most important are: the development of relatively safe, readily applicable angiographic techniques, which permit precise delineation of the location, nature and extent of disease in the heart and arterial system; development of highly successful surgical procedures for vascular replacement (with restoration of normal circulation or replacement of the excised diseased segment with an arterial substitute); and a tremendous surge of interest in and intensification of investigative endeavors, undoubtedly a result of the initially successful surgery on some cardiovascular problems that had long seemed hopeless.

Although the era of modern cardiovascular surgery may be considered to be the past three or four decades, certain developments preceding this period are not only of historical interest, but also help to provide a better appreciation of subsequent events. The idea of suturing blood vessels was conceived more than two centuries ago by an Englishman named Lambert who suggested the method to his colleague, Mr. Hallowell. On June 15, 1759, Hallowell successfully applied it to an artery in a patient's arm which had been punctured for therapeutic bleeding—a popular treatment for various illnesses at the time. Further efforts in this direction, however, were soon discouraged, particularly because of the unsuccessful experiments of Conrad Asman of Groningen, in the Netherlands, in 1773, and the technique of suturing blood vessels fell into disuse for more than a century. Additional factors, which may have contributed to the decline of work along these lines, were the prestige accorded the Hunterian ligature following its development in 1785 and the dominant concepts of Antonio Scarpa regarding the healing of aneurysms. John Hunter was one of the great English surgeons and investigators who devised the principle of treating aneurysms of the arteries in the limbs by a single ligature applied to the healthy part of the artery, well above the aneurysm. Antonio Scarpa, a great and influential Italian surgeon and anatomist who lived in the late eighteenth and early nineteenth centuries, stated that " . . . a complete and radical cure of aneurysm cannot be obtained . . . unless the ulcerated, lacerated, or wounded artery from which the aneurysm is derived is, by the assistance of nature or of nature combined with art, obliterated and converted into a perfectly solid ligamentous substance. . . ."

Interest in vascular suturing was revived toward the latter part of the nineteenth century, probably because of the impetus given to experimental surgery by the Listerian doctrine which provided a sterile environment and greatly reduced the incidence of infection, a previously grave complication. Further interest in vascular suturing was stimulated in 1881 by its successful application in a patient with an injured internal jugular vein by Vincenz Czerny of Germany and by Dr. P. Postempski in Italy, five years later, in a lateral wound of the femoral artery. The development of endoaneurysmorrhaphy (obliteration of the lumen of an aneurysm by suturing together the inner wall and all openings into it) in 1888 by Rudolph Matas, one of the great American pioneers in vascular surgery, was a tremendous impetus to the revival of interest in the suture of blood vessels; it provided the first successful challenge to the "law laid down by Scarpa" more than one hundred years earlier. In 1889, Alexander Jassinowsky of Germany performed a series of experiments demonstrating the successful suturing of blood vessels.

The next few decades witnessed intense investigative activity in this field, both in America and abroad, distinguished by the work of a number of surgeons, including Nikolai Eck, J. B. Murphy, Julius Dörfler, Erwin Payr, Alexis Carrel, C. C. Guthrie, E. Bode, E. Fabian, and Alexander Jassinowsky. At the turn of the century several researchers, particularly Drs. Alexis Carrel and C. C. Guthrie, had clearly demonstrated in experimental animals the feasibility of excising arterial segments and restoring continuity by end-to-end anastomosis, or by use of arterial grafts, as well as organ transplants, such as the kidney and heart. A few patients with aneurysms or injuries of peripheral arteries had been treated by these methods with some success. In 1896, John Benjamin Murphy of Chicago, after establishing the success of the procedure in a series of experiments, resected about one-half inch of a patient's femoral artery that had been lacerated by a bullet, and sutured the ends together. In 1906, Dr. D. José Goyanes of Spain reported the successful excision of an aneurysm of the popliteal artery with restoration of continuity by grafting a vein. The following year, Professor Erich Lexer, in Germany, reported a similar successful operation in the axillary artery.

Except for the individual efforts of a few surgeons at the time, little consideration was given to the application of these principles in the treatment of aortic disease. In 1902, for example, Professor Marin Théodore Tuffier of Paris reported an unsuccessful case of ligation of the neck or opening of the aneurysm in a patient with a sacciform aneurysm of the ascending aorta, but this experience convinced him of the feasibility of excisional therapy with lateral repair by suture. The foresight of some of these early scientists is further illustrated by another pioneering French surgeon, Professor René Leriche, who predicted in 1923 that the ideal treatment for occlusive disease of the abdominal aorta (since termed Leriche's syndrome) would be excision of the diseased segment and its replacement with an aortic graft. About fifty years elapsed before Tuffier's recommendation was put into practice, and it was thirty years before Leriche's prediction became a reality. A number of factors contributed to this delay. For one thing, certain ancillary surgical measures, particularly methods for inducing anesthesia, blood transfusion and chemotherapy or antibiotic therapy, had not developed adequately enough to support extensive vascular procedures. For another, the specialty of surgery had not matured sufficiently to accept such an aggressive approach to complex surgical problems. Finally, arteriography, an important diagnostic procedure for precisely identifying the type and location of arterial lesions, had not yet been developed.

The interest in vascular surgery was probably revived initially in 1944, by successful treatment of coarctation of the aorta (by excision and repair through end-to-end anastomosis) by Clarence Crafoord in Sweden and Robert Gross in Boston. A few years later Drs. Robert Gross and Charles Hufnagel reported the successful repair, with aortic homografts, of the defect in the aorta resulting from excision of coarctation in cases in which the ends could not be approximated. Considerable impetus was thus given to further development of these approaches to treatment of arterial lesions, leading to renewed interest in using homografts to bridge excised segments, thereby permitting broader application of this method to other aortic lesions. In 1951, J. Oudot, in Paris, treated the first case of occlusive disease of the lower abdominal aorta by excision and replacement with a homograft, as originally recommended by René Leriche almost thirty years earlier. In the next year,

Dr. Charles Dubost of Paris, and shortly afterward, Dr. Michael DeBakey, successfully performed the procedure for aneurysm of the abdominal aorta. In 1953, Dr. DeBakey also performed the first successful case of resection of a fusiform aneurysm of the thoracic aorta with restoration of continuity by an aortic homograft (Figure 38), and in the following year, did the first

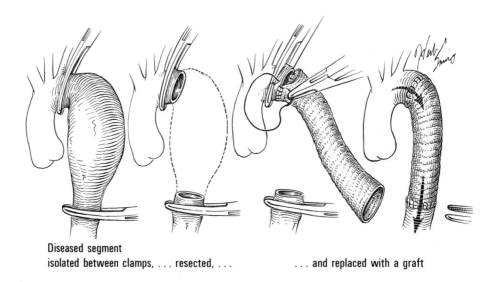

Diseased segment
isolated between clamps, . . . resected, ... and replaced with a graft

Figure 38. Technique for resection of diseased segment of artery and graft replacement

successful resection of an aneurysm of the distal aortic arch and of a dissecting aneurysm of the descending thoracic aorta. During the next few years, this method of surgical excision and graft replacement was also first successfully used by Dr. DeBakey in the treatment of aneurysms of the ascending aorta, the thoraco-abdominal segment, and the entire aortic arch. Thus, within a decade, excisional therapy of aortic lesions had become a reality, and the age-old challenge had been successfully met.

During this early period, aortic and arterial homografts (removed from cadavers) were used to replace the excised diseased segments, and although they functioned satisfactorily, they had a number of disadvantages, the most important being their limited availability and the inconvenience of their procurement, sterilization and preservation. Later studies also indicated that the tissue elements of the graft gradually deteriorated and lead to complications. For these reasons, about 1951, Dr. DeBakey, as well as a number of other investigators, directed their efforts toward development of an arterial substitute that had none of these disadvantages. Various materials, such as nylon, Ivalon, Orlon, Teflon, and Dacron, were fashioned into tubes by different methods, including heat-sealing, sewing, braiding, knitting and weaving. Extensive experiments in our laboratory showed that Dacron had

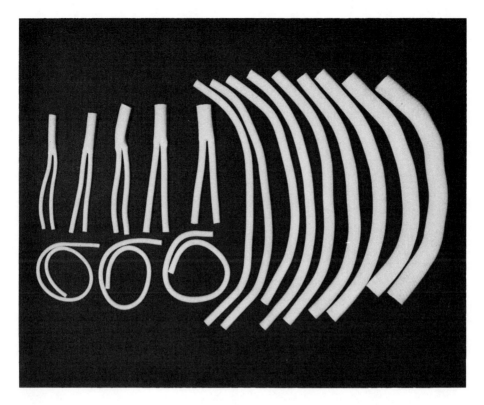

Figure 39. Dacron vascular grafts

the most desirable characteristics for this purpose. With the assistance of Professor Thomas Edman of Philadelphia, a textile expert, a new knitting machine was designed and built to produce seamless knitted Dacron tubes in different sizes and in the form of bifurcations (Figure 39). An important feature of this Dacron arterial substitute is its porosity, which permits the blood to seep through its wall until sufficient clotting has occurred in the interstices of the fabric to seal it and thus prevent further leakage of blood. This porosity also permits subsequent ingrowth of tissue to produce firm attachment of the new intima lining the inner surface. In other words, the body builds its own new tissue around the Dacron fabric and thus creates a new artery. Our experience with these Dacron grafts as arterial substitutes for a variety of aortic and arterial diseases in more than 30,000 patients has been extremely gratifying. Follow-up studies extending over a period of more than two decades have shown that the long-term function of these grafts is excellent. We have many patients with functioning grafts even after twenty years. There is every reason to believe that these grafts should last the entire lifetime of the patient. Late failure of the graft may occur, but this is usually due to exacerbation of the disease in the artery distal to the anastomosis. The resulting decrease in blood flow through the graft may be sufficient to precipitate clotting in much the same way as when this occurs in the diseased artery.

During the past decade, Dr. DeBakey designed a new type of Dacron graft, which was an outgrowth of our experimental work on the artificial heart. Efforts to find a better lining for these pumps led to the development of a velour fabric, which had the advantage of providing firm adherence of the new inner lining. This observation led us to experiment with velour as an arterial substitute. The Dacron velour fabric is warp-knitted in such a way that loops of yarn are extended almost perpendicular to the fabric surface (Figure 40). This produces the velvety appearance that one sees on the inner

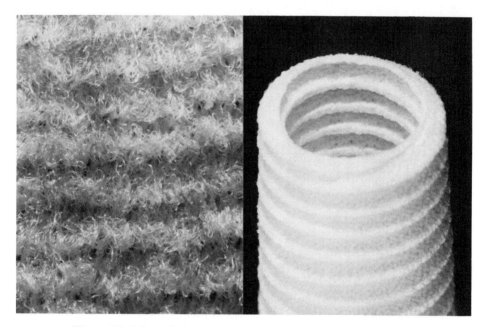

Figure 40. Magnified view (left) of velour fabric used to line interior of Dacron vascular grafts (right)

surface of the graft. The fibrin and circulating cells are trapped and become firmly attached to these loops. The ingrowth of tissue is better and more adherent to this velour surface. When laboratory experiments demonstrated these advantages, we used the graft in patients, and now, after experience with more than one thousand cases, it has proved to be a further improvement on previously used Dacron grafts.

In devising endarterectomy in 1947, Professor J. Cid dos Santos of Lisbon, Portugal, whose father performed the first abdominal aortography, made another important contribution to vascular surgery. After observing that certain forms of atherosclerosis could be easily peeled away from the remaining arterial wall, he reasoned that this might constitute the basis for surgical treatment. In certain forms of atherosclerosis the plaquelike lesion is well localized, with normal artery above and below it. This can be determined precisely by arteriography (radiographic visualization of the lumen of the artery after injection of a radiopaque material). The procedure consists of applying occluding clamps to the artery above and below the lesion, and then making a longitudinal incision through the arterial wall and the occluding lesion into the normal wall immediately above and below the lesion (Figure 41). A proper cleavage plane is then found at the base of the lesion, and it is carefully separated and peeled away from the remaining arterial wall with a blunt-ended instrument in much the same way as one would peel the skin of an orange. After the atheromatous plaque has been

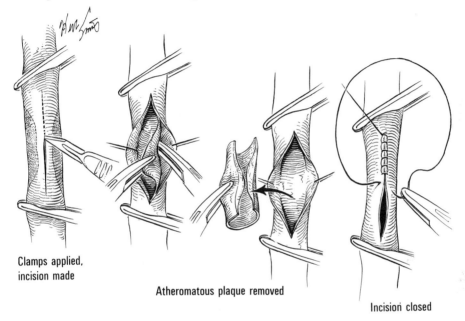

Clamps applied,
incision made

Atheromatous plaque removed

Incision closed

Figure 41. Technique for removing atherosclerotic lesion by endarterectomy

completely removed, the edges of the remaining arterial wall are sewed together, and blood flow through this new lumen is restored by removal of the occluding clamps. The procedure was rapidly and widely adopted by vascular surgeons, and has proved to be eminently successful when properly applied.

Another contribution in this area was the development of patch graft angioplasty by Dr. DeBakey. It was observed that after completion of endarterectomy, closure of the incision in the arterial wall sometimes necessitated use of some of the circumference of the arterial wall and caused narrowing of the resulting lumen. To overcome this, a patch of Dacron fabric, or a small segment of vein that was slit open, was inserted between the two edges of the artery and sutured in place (Figure 42). This provided an

excellent method of repairing the opening in the artery without narrowing
the lumen. We later found this method useful in certain types of arterial
disease in which the lumen was narrowed, but in which endarterectomy was
not indicated; the narrowed arterial segment could thus be widened by use of
such a patch graft and blood flow restored through a normal lumen.

Still another important contribution to vascular surgery was made by
Professor J. Kunlin of France, with whom Dr. DeBakey had the good fortune
to be associated as a foreign assistant working under Professor René Leriche
at the University of Strasbourg. Professor Kunlin observed that certain forms
of occlusive disease in the arteries of the leg were well localized and that

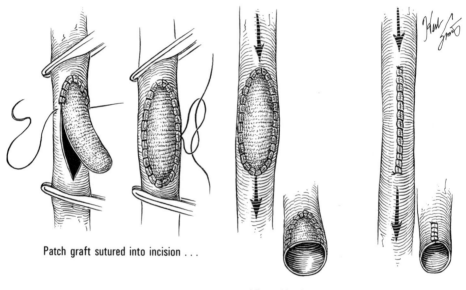

Patch graft sutured into incision . . .

. . . providing wider lumen . . .   . . . than direct closure

Figure 42. Technique for patch-graft angioplasty

beyond the diseased segment the artery was normal. Circulation to the leg
beyond the obstructed segment was maintained through small collateral
communications, which is nature's way of trying to overcome the decreased
circulation produced by the obstructed arterial segment. Circulation through
these small vessels may be adequate to maintain viability, but it is often not
enough to maintain normal function. On this basis, Professor Kunlin
reasoned that it should be possible to aid nature's efforts to restore circulation
around the obstructed segment by attaching a graft (using a segment of vein
taken from the leg) to an opening in the side of the normal artery above the
obstructed segment, and then, in similar fashion, to the normal artery below
the obstructed segment (Figure 43). In this way blood would be shunted
through the graft around the obstructed segment, and thus normal circula-

tion would be restored. For this reason the operation is referred to as a bypass graft. In 1949, Professor Kunlin reported successful performance of this procedure on a patient suffering from a circulatory problem in the leg due to

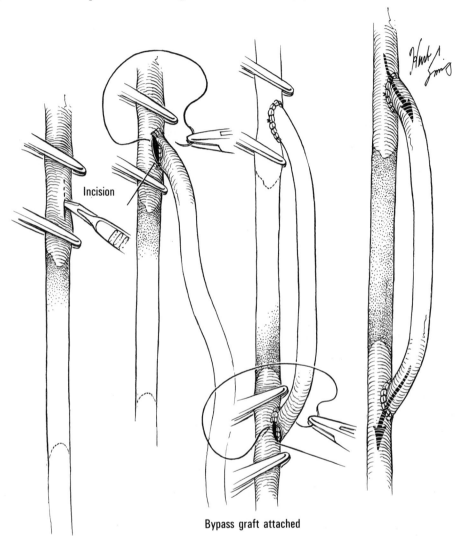

Incision

Bypass graft attached

Figure 43. Technique for bypass graft to shunt blood around diseased segment of artery

occlusion of the femoral artery. Since then, this method has been widely and effectively used to restore circulation for various types of occlusive disease.

One of the most important contributions to cardiovascular surgery was the development of angiography, which provided the underlying basis for many brilliant achievements in this field. This diagnostic procedure made possible the radiographic visualization and precise delineation of diseases of the heart and blood vessels. It also established the fact that many arterial lesions are well localized to one segment, with relatively normal arteries above and below the lesion and, therefore, are amenable to direct surgical treatment.

Radiographic visualization of the blood vessels became a reality shortly after the monumental discovery of x-rays by Wilhelm Konrad Roentgen of Germany, in 1895. Within a month of this breakthrough, scientists began experimenting with its potential clinical applications, for such ailments as bone fractures. In January 1896, E. Von Haschek and O. Th. Lindenthal of Germany injected a *radiopaque* substance into the blood vessels of an amputated hand and thus first demonstrated the feasibility of radiographic visualization of blood vessels. The potential diagnostic value of this procedure fired the imagination of a number of medical scientists. The major problem that limited the clinical application of this method was the need for an injectable, nontoxic, radiopaque substance. This problem proved difficult to resolve, and indeed, it was not until 1923 that the next major advances occurred. Two French scientists, J. A. Sicard and J. Forestier, using Lipiodol, an oil iodine mixture which they had developed to visualize the bronchial tree on the x-ray, injected the mixture into a patient's femoral vein and watched it on the fluoroscope proceed to the heart and then to the lungs. In the same year, two German scientists, Drs. J. Berberich and S. Hirsch, developed a bromide solution which they used to demonstrate arteriography and venography for the first time in a living man. The next year, Barney Brooks, an American surgeon, showed that injection of sodium iodide provided good visualization of the arteries of the lower limbs, was useful in visualizing atheromatous disease of the arteries, and could indicate when amputation was necessary.

The early twentieth century was an exciting developmental period for angiography. Medical scientists from many parts of the world were eagerly pursuing this unique and precise diagnostic procedure. The Portuguese medical scientists proved to be pioneers in this endeavor. Egas Moniz, a Portuguese neurosurgeon, devised the technique of carotid arteriography to visualize the arteries of the brain, and later angiopneumography to visualize the pulmonary vessels. R. dos Santos of Lisbon developed translumbar aortography, a method still used today but with much safer radiopaque solutions. Although the technical feasibility and diagnostic value of arteriography had been demonstrated by then, the injectible solutions used were still not satisfactory; they were often irritating and produced other undesirable complications. The substance needed would provide good radiographic visualization but produce no negative reactions. An important breakthrough toward this objective came in 1929, when Dr. M. Swick of Germany reported the successful use of an organic iodide solution developed by two German scientists, A. Bing and C. Roth. This stimulated several workers to synthesize other radiopaque drugs which finally led to highly effective and safe injectible solutions like those used today.

Cardioangiography and cardiac catheterization were also major developments that significantly influenced cardiac surgery. This began in 1928 with the experiments of Werner Forssmann of Germany, who became intrigued with the idea of cardiac catheterization as a means of injecting therapeutic drugs directly into the heart. Working on cadavers, he easily inserted a catheter into a vein in the arm and moved it into the right atrium. He did the first clinical experiment on himself. Using a fine catheter ordinarily used for urologic purposes, he inserted the catheter through a wide-bore needle into one of the veins in his arm with the aid of an assistant. As the catheter approached the heart, his assistant became so fearful that he refused to continue, and the trial ended. But with the firm conviction of a dedicated scientist, Forssmann decided to proceed by himself a week later. After inserting the catheter through a vein in his arm and pushing it into his right atrium, he walked a distance, upstairs, to the x-ray room, and radiographically confirmed the location of the catheter. Later, using this same technique, he injected a radiopaque substance through the catheter into his right atrium and obtained a roentgenogram of the cardiac chambers. During the next decade, a number of investigators from different parts of the world contributed to its development, particularly Drs. André Cournand and Dickinson W. Richards, who, with Forssman, received the Nobel Prize in 1956. Others, such as Drs. P. Rosthoi of Sweden, P. Amenille of France, A. Castellanos of Cuba, and G. P. Robb, I. Steinberg and F. M. Sones of the United States, added further significant improvements and refinements to the technique, thus making it a versatile diagnostic method applicable to all forms of cardiovascular disease.

Medical history abounds with pioneering surgical developments stimulated by military or civilian injuries. This is particularly true of some of the early surgical procedures on the heart. In the early nineteenth century, Baron Larrey, who was Napoleon's great military surgeon, successfully drained blood and fluid from the pericardial sac around the heart. In 1896, Ludwig Rehn, a German surgeon, successfully sutured a penetrating wound of the heart, and thus defied the erroneous prediction by a distinguished English surgeon, Stephen Paget, who had just written that " . . . surgery of the heart has probably reached the limits set by nature to all surgery." In 1903, Professor Marin Théodore Tuffier, a famous French surgeon, removed a bullet which had lodged in the wall of the left atrium. During World War II, Dwight Harken, a distinguished American surgeon, demonstrated the feasibility of removing retained foreign bodies in the heart, and thus provided another illustration of how the surgery of trauma inspired further advances.

The first cardiac operation, exclusive of traumatic cases, was performed by a French surgeon, Edmond Delorme, in 1898, for an infection of the pericardium. In 1902, Sir Lauder Bronton advocated surgical treatment for mitral stenosis, but more than two decades elapsed before his suggestion was followed. In the meantime, two French surgeons attempted to dilate stenosed heart valves. In 1913, Eugene Doyen attempted to dilate a stenotic pulmonary valve, and one year later, Marin Théodore Tuffier made a similar attempt on the aortic valve, but with little success. In 1923, Elliott Cutler and S. A. Levine of Boston devised a special valvulotome, which could be inserted into the chamber of the heart to cut the mitral valve. They performed this operation on a few patients with limited success. Two years later, Sir Henry S. Souttar, an English surgeon, inserted his left forefinger through an opening in the left atrium to feel the stenosed mitral valve, but found that it was already dilated, and decided not to section the valve. Although convinced of the feasibility of the procedure, he later complained that he could get no other case " . . . as medical opinion was solidly against such attempts." It was not until the late 1940s that further attempts along these lines were revived by Dwight Harken of Boston, Charles Bailey of Philadelphia, and Lord Brock of London. The great interest stimulated by their success led other surgeons to make technical improvements in the operation, and within a few years, the procedures were widely adopted for certain forms of mitral and pulmonic stenosis.

Although as early as 1907, John Munro of Boston had proposed tying off a patent ductus *arteriosus*, the treatment for congenital abnormalities of the heart remained ineffective until 1937, when Ashton Graybiel, John Strieder, and N. H. Boyer of Boston made an unsuccessful attempt to ligate a patent ductus arteriosus. The next year, however, Robert Gross of Boston performed the procedure successfully, and thus initiated great interest in the surgical attack upon certain congenital anomalies. This was further enhanced by the successful surgical treatment of coarctation of the aorta by Clarence Crafoord of Stockholm in 1944, and Robert Gross shortly thereafter. Additional impetus was provided by the successful "blue baby" operation by Alfred Blalock and Helen Taussig of Baltimore in 1945. This consisted of anastomosing the subclavian artery to the pulmonary artery, in order to increase the blood flow through the lung and thereby obtain a higher blood oxygen content.

Congenital defects, such as patent ductus arteriosus and coarctation of the aorta, were amenable to surgical correction because the surgeon was operating on blood vessels outside of the heart. Beyond these abnormalities were all those congenital and acquired cardiac diseases and injuries that could be corrected only by opening the heart. Until a safe way to open the heart could be discovered, the vast range of cardiac diseases lay beyond the surgeon's skill.

The primary obstacle to further progress was the need to maintain circulation of the blood to the rest of the body, particularly to the brain with its need for a constant supply of oxygenated blood, while interrupting the work of the heart for a few hours. The brain will survive only about four minutes without permanent damage if its supply of oxygenated blood is blocked.

To gain sufficient operating time, surgeons experimented with *hypo-thermia*, a procedure in which the patient is packed in ice or wrapped in refrigerated blankets to cool the body well below the normal temperature. Experiments on animals had shown that hypothermia reduced cardiac output, pulse rate, blood pressure, and oxygen consumption. Cells, including those of the brain, survive longer when chilled.

But cooling and then warming the body often resulted in serious adverse effects. In some patients, ventricular fibrillation developed—instead of the muscle fibers of the heart uniting in coordinated contraction and relaxation, a rapid flutter of separate muscle strands occurred. The dispersion of effort by heart muscle that is too weak to pump blood causes immediate death.

The possibility of extracorporeal circulation, that is, circulating the patient's blood outside the body to keep it supplied with oxygen while stopping the pumping of the heart, became the objective of intense research. Such a mechanical device would need to perform two complicated functions: the steady pumping of blood that did not damage delicate cells, and adequate oxygenation. Efforts to construct such a machine date back to 1885. For a brief time, scientists toyed with the idea of using a lung removed from an animal and aerated by artificial respiration to oxygenate blood, but that approach was considered unsuitable for humans. Others experimented and a few actually used a human donor temporarily connected to the patient for cross circulation, but none of these methods proved a satisfactory solution to the problem.

In the United States, the development of the heart-lung machine owes much to the pioneering work of John Gibbon of Philadelphia. In 1931, while a resident in a Boston hospital, he treated a fifty-three-year-old woman dying from a series of blood clots that blocked her pulmonary artery. In a letter to a friend, Gibbon recalled, "During the seventeen hours by this patient's side, the thought constantly recurred that the patient's hazardous condition could be improved if some of the blue blood in the patient's distended veins could be continuously withdrawn into an apparatus where the blood could pick up oxygen and discharge carbon dioxide and then be pumped back into the patient's arteries. Such a procedure would also lend support to the patient's circulation while the embolectomy (removal of the clots) was performed." During an emergency operation on the woman, the surgeon removed the emboli in only six and one-half minutes, but the patient died on the operating table, for lack of a life-supporting system such as Gibbon described.

Three years later, Gibbon began to design a heart-lung machine at the Massachusetts General Hospital. He reminisced, "I bought an air pump in a second-hand shop in East Boston for a few dollars, and used it to activate the ... blood pumps." To test his apparatus, he experimented with cats. "When our supply ran short, I can recall prowling around Beacon Hill at night with some tuna fish as bait and a gunnysack to catch one of the numerous stray alley cats which swarmed over Boston in those days."

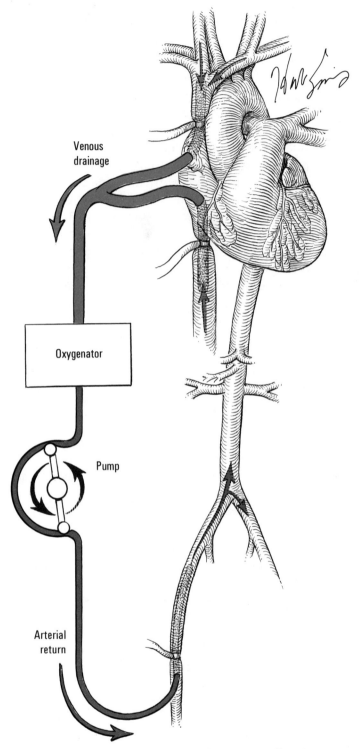

Venous
drainage

Oxygenator

Pump

Arterial
return

Figure 44. The heart-lung machine, or cardiopulmonary
bypass, oxygenates the venous blood from the patient and
then pumps it throughout the arterial system.

Gibbon eventually proved that animals could survive thirty to forty minutes of complete bypass of their own hearts and lungs while supported by his machine. Most of his cats died, however, a few hours after their own circulation was restored. Apparently, the pumping mechanism seriously damaged blood cells, producing fatal clots.

During this period, Dr. DeBakey designed a roller pump to facilitate direct transfusions of blood from donor to patient. This pump's rollers moved blood without injury to it. DeBakey suggested to Gibbon that he try this pump, which he then installed in his machine and found to be highly effective. Since then, it has become the standard pump for heart-lung machines. Still, the oxygenation process seemed to be insufficient for the needs of an animal, to say nothing of a human. World War II delayed further research, but in 1945 Gibbon resumed work on his project. He convinced International Business Machines to assign some of its technicians and engineers to help him construct a heart-lung machine.

In 1950, about nineteen years after his initial effort to develop a life-supporting mechanical system outside of the human body, Gibbon decided his machine was ready for use. His first patient, a fifteen-month-old baby, died shortly after the operation. Instead of the atrial defect originally diagnosed, the infant had been a victim of a large patent ductus. Gibbon's second attempt on May 6, 1954, was on an eighteen-year-old girl with an atrial septal defect. The heart-lung machine functioned beautifully, and the operation was a total success. It would seem that the feasibility of the total heart-lung bypass had been proved, and this encouraged others to perfect the oxygenating component of the machine.

The principle of the heart-lung machine, or, as it is termed medically, cardiopulmonary bypass, is relatively simple (Figure 44). It consists essentially of diverting all the venous blood returning to the heart to the artificial lung of the heart-lung machine, where oxygen is added and carbon dioxide is removed. The refreshed blood is then pumped into the arterial system of the patient. In this way, the function of the heart and lungs is temporarily assumed by the machine. Thus, life-supporting circulation is provided to the rest of the body while certain types of corrective surgical procedures are performed within the heart or on one of its vessels. The procedure is usually performed by inserting two plastic cannulas through the wall of the right atrium into the upper and lower venae cavae, the two major veins returning blood to the heart. By encircling and tightening two cotton tapes placed around the venae cavae and around the inserted plastic tubes, all blood from the venae cavae is shunted into the heart-lung machine. After passing through the artificial lung, the blood is returned to the patient, by means of the pump, through a plastic tube inserted into one of the major arteries in the groin or into the ascending aorta. Some variations in this procedure may be necessary, depending upon the patient's condition and specific problems.

7

CONGENITAL
ABNORMALITIES
OF THE HEART

THE first major cardiovascular disorders to yield to treatment were congenital defects, and their repair required surgical correction. To comprehend what was involved requires knowledge of the evolution of the heart, from conception to birth.

Toward the end of the first month of fetal life, the heart begins to develop (Figure 45). After about four more weeks a fully developed tiny replica of an adult heart has formed. The process starts with a group of cells organizing themselves into a hollow tube; one end is called the venous and the other, the arterial. The tube grows faster than the space around it. Under the pressure of confinement, the tube bends, first into a U and then an S shape. The venous end bulges into a pocket which eventually will form both the right and left atria.

Meanwhile, the middle section of the original hollow tube expands into a bag shape which will form the right and left ventricles; clumps of cells arrange themselves into the vital mitral and tricuspid valves.

At the arterial end of the original hollow tube, another division occurs. A

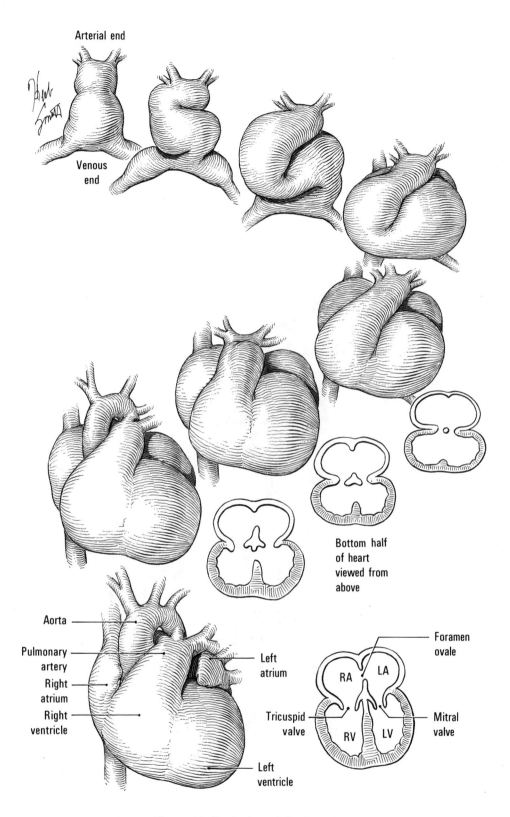

Arterial end

Venous end

Bottom half of heart viewed from above

Aorta

Pulmonary artery

Right atrium

Right ventricle

Left atrium

Left ventricle

Foramen ovale

RA   LA

Tricuspid valve

Mitral valve

RV   LV

Figure 45. Evolution of the fetal heart

partition separates the once single trunk into two channels: the aorta and the pulmonary artery. Obeying the genetic instructions for human embryonic development, other cells dutifully build the tissue of the aortic and pulmonary valves.

A bare two months after conception, the fetal heart looks like an adult heart, but a major portion of its functions remain dependent upon the mother. This continues even after it begins to beat during the later stages of pregnancy. The oxygenation of blood to feed the growing tissue of the fetus, and the elimination of waste occur in the mother's placenta (Figure 46).

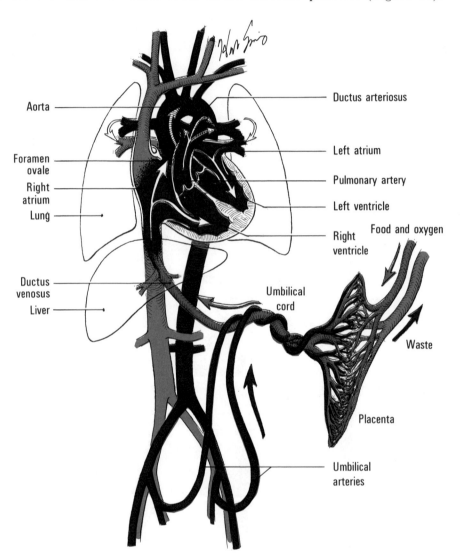

Figure 46. During pregnancy, the mother's placenta provides oxygen and food to the fetal circulation and eliminates the wastes from the fetus.

Oxygenated blood passes through the umbilical cord into the fetus' *ductus venosus,* a vessel that bypasses the unborn's liver and leads directly to the inferior vena cava and hence to the right atrium. Unlike a normal adult, whose blood in the right atrium lacks oxygen, the fetus collects oxygenated blood into this chamber from the inferior vena cava. Because of the *foramen ovale* (the opening between the atria), some of the oxygenated blood in the right atrium flows into the left atrium. The remaining blood in the right atrium conventionally enters the right ventricle and is pumped out into the pulmonary arteries during systole. But instead of flowing the length of the

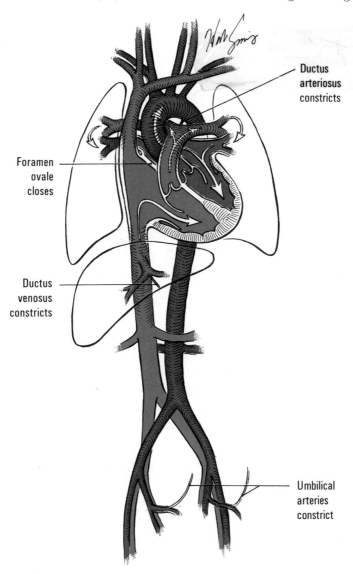

Ductus
arteriosus
constricts

Foramen
ovale
closes

Ductus
venosus
constricts

Umbilical
arteries
constrict

Figure 47. At birth the infant's circulatory system becomes self-sufficient.

pulmonary artery, most of the blood is diverted before it reaches the lungs into the *ductus arteriosus,* a fetal blood vessel that connects the pulmonary artery with the aorta. The fetal lungs, which do not breathe while inside the womb, require only enough blood to nourish the growing tissue. Meanwhile, the oxygenated blood, flowing through the foramen ovale into the left atrium, reaches the left ventricle and is pumped out into the aorta.

At birth the infant develops a new circulatory system (Figure 47). As the baby begins to breathe, the ductus arteriosus constricts, thus closing the communication between the pulmonary artery and the aorta. Unused, the ductus arteriosus normally degenerates into a solid cord of tissue called the ligamentum arteriosum. Now blood pumped from the right ventricle can flow only into the lungs. It returns to the left side of the heart through the pulmonary veins. During contraction of the heart, the left atrium exerts hydraulic pressure which prevents the flow of any blood from the right atrium into the left. The foramen ovale is so constructed that this continued high pressure in the left atrium over the period of a year turns the foramen ovale into a flap that seals the prenatal opening. The ductus venosus, the original pipeline from the mother's placenta, also loses its function and turns into a ligament across the lower half of the child's liver.

This complicated mechanism of cellular growth and organization characterizes the development of every human heart. Whereas any manufacturer would be delighted with the remarkably high rate of flawless units that mark human reproduction, the small percentage of imperfections (less than one per thousand) poses grave threats to the lives of those with such congenital heart defects.

Patent Ductus Arteriosus

The first human congenital cardiac defect to be corrected surgically was patent ductus arteriosus, the fetal vessel between the pulmonary artery and the aorta that fails to close (Figure 48). Some researchers believe that German measles in the mother during the early months of pregnancy may cause this condition which heightens pressure in the pulmonary artery. A second threat of patent ductus seems to be that bacterial infection often develops around the defect.

Symptoms produced by the lesion vary depending upon the size of the ductus and the amount of blood shunted from the aorta into the pulmonary artery. Most patients with the condition tire more quickly than normal infants. Often the disorder retards growth and heart failure may also occur. Usually diagnosis can easily be made soon after birth by a characteristic murmur.

As early as 1907, Dr. John Munro of Boston proposed a procedure to tie off, or ligate, a patent ductus. He had worked extensively on cadavers, but surgeons were reluctant to attempt the operation on their patients because the diagnosis could not be made with certainty by the available methods at the time. After adequate research had been done to clearly identify the syndrome of patent ductus, a new assault on the defect began. In 1938, a young surgical resident at Boston Children's Hospital, Robert Gross, successfully ligated a seven-year-old girl's patent ductus with a single-braid

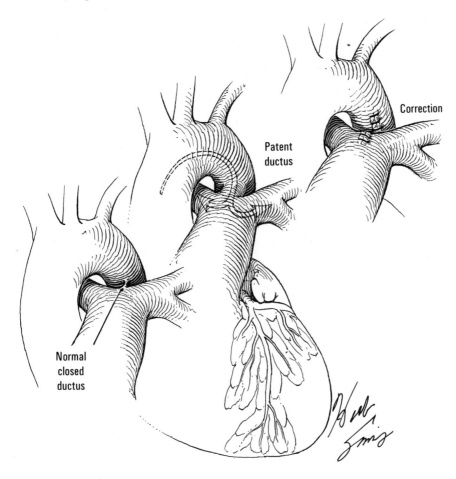

Figure 48. Patent ductus arteriosis resulting from failure of normal closure after birth of fetal connection between the aorta and pulmonary artery

silk suture. This feat convinced surgeons that the condition could be corrected by surgery.

If left uncorrected, a patent ductus can lead to serious complications and early death in the majority of patients. Even if the infant survives the early period of life, pulmonary vascular resistance may take place causing the condition to become inoperable. For this reason, and because the risk of operation is virtually zero if performed within the first few years of life, surgical correction is the only effective therapy. The procedure consists essentially of division and suture closure (Figure 48).

Coarctation of the Thoracic Aorta

The second congenital abnormality to yield to surgical repair was *coarctation of the aorta*, a severe narrowing of the great artery, usually in the arch where the bloodstream divides to service both the upper and lower parts of the body (Figure 49). Coarctation causes high blood pressure because the

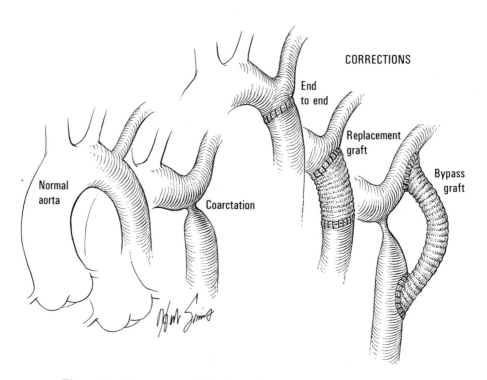

Figure 49. Coarctation of the thoracic aorta consists of severe narrowing of lumen, causing obstruction to blood flow.

heart must pump harder to provide adequate circulation beyond the narrowed segment. Victims of coarctation usually do not live longer than fifty years unless the condition is corrected. Again, a long period of experimentation on animals and cadavers preceded any attempts at correction on humans. The simplest and most attractive approach consisted of clamping the aorta on both sides of the constriction. The constricted section could then be removed and the two ends of the aorta stretched together and sutured. In 1944, this procedure was sucessfully performed on a twelve-year-old boy with coarctation by Dr. Clarence Crafoord of Sweden.

The human body makes a valiant effort to compensate for a disorder such as coarctation of the aorta. Blood vessels branching off the subclavian arteries in the upper half of the body enlarge and communicate with other arteries to provide some circulation to regions below the point of coarctation. Because of this collateral circulation, symptoms of coarctation may not appear early in life, and for some patients the condition goes unnoticed through young adulthood.

Early surgical correction of coarctation is recommended and, ideally, should be done between the ages of eight and twelve, when the aorta has grown to provide a lumen of sufficient size for subsequent growth of the

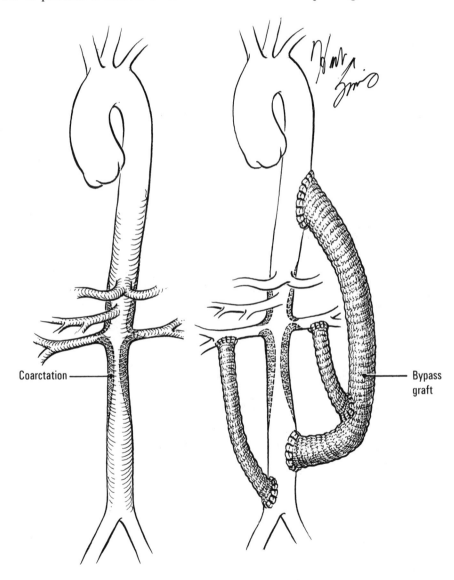

Figure 50. Coarctation of the abdominal aorta

patient. Today, surgical correction consists essentially of excising the coarctated segment and reconnecting the two ends or by replacing the segment with a Dacron graft. In some older patients it may be preferable to use a bypass graft. In uncomplicated forms of coarcation the risk of operation is very low—about 1 or 2 percent—and the results are excellent.

Coarctation of the Abdominal Aorta

Although coarctation of the aorta usually affects the thoracic aorta as described above, occasionally it may involve other segments of the aorta, particularly the abdominal aorta, affecting the origins of the major arteries to the abdominal arteries (Figure 50). It has been estimated that this type of coarctation occurs in about 2 percent of the cases. It seems to occur more commonly in females in a ratio of about three or four to one and becomes apparent at an early age, with most cases being diagnosed during the first two decades of life.

Among the most important signs and symptoms of the condition are severe hypertension (high blood pressure), headache, fatigue after minimal exercise and decreased blood pressure in the lower extremities. If untreated, the prognosis is poor, with eventual death from heart failure or cerebral hemorrhage.

Treatment is surgical and consists of placing a bypass graft from the descending thoracic aorta to the abdominal aorta. Since most cases have involvement of the renal arteries, it is usually necessary to place additional bypass grafts to these arteries. Occasionally it is also necessary to perform bypasses to the celiac and superior mesenteric arteries.

Results of operation are excellent. In our experience, there have been no deaths and all patients responded favorably, with restoration of normal or near normal blood pressure, and were able to assume normal activities.

Anomalies of the Aortic Arch Causing Vascular Rings

In the embryological development of the aortic arch, certain abnormalities may occur that result in *vascular rings* which surround the esophagus and trachea and may produce symptoms of obstruction (Figure 51). Among the most common of the several varieties of this abnormality are the double aortic arch and the right aortic arch associated with a segment passing behind the esophagus and a left-sided ligamentum arteriosum. Many patients with this type of abnormality remain asymptomatic and appear to lead a normal life. Under the circumstances, no treatment is necessary. In those who develop symptoms, these usually occur in infancy or early life and are manifested by noisy respiration, difficulty in swallowing and repeated pulmonary infections. Under these circumstances, surgery is recommended and consists of dividing and ligating, or closing, the ends of the smaller of the

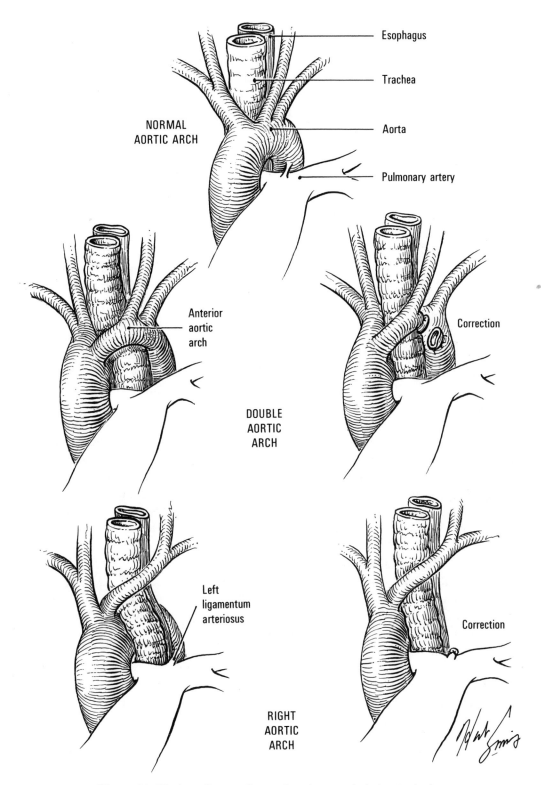

Figure 51. Various forms of vascular rings and their surgical corrections

Labels in figure:

NORMAL
AORTIC ARCH

Esophagus

Trachea

Aorta

Pulmonary artery

Anterior
aortic
arch

DOUBLE
AORTIC
ARCH

Correction

Left
ligamentum
arteriosus

Correction

RIGHT
AORTIC
ARCH

two aortic arches or of the left-sided ligamentum arteriosum. Results of operation are excellent, with little or no risk.

Tetralogy of Fallot

In 1888, a French physician, Étienne-Louis Arthur Fallot, described a four-fold congenital malady of the heart, tetralogy of Fallot, which bears his name. Although four separate problems are recognized in this condition, the primary defects consist of a stenosis-narrowed pulmonary valve and an opening in the septum wall between the ventricles (Figure 52). The defective valve prevents an adequate amount of blood from being pumped through the pulmonary artery to the lungs, and the hole in the septum permits unoxygenated blood to mix with the normally oxygenated supply in the left ventricle. As a result, the child receives a grossly inadequate supply of oxygenated blood, a condition often manifested by a bluish tinge called cyanosis—a sign that has popularized the abnormality as the blue baby disease. Apart from the bluish tinge, symptoms of the malformation include clubbing of fingernails and toenails, particularly as the child grows older, labored breathing, frequent fatigue and stunted growth.

Dr. Helen Taussig conceived of the approach to correct this defect. In charge of a cardiac clinic at Johns Hopkins Hospital in Baltimore at the time, she noticed that children with tetralogy of Fallot actually fared better if they also had a patent ductus arteriosus. From this observation she deduced that the patent ductus supplemented the supply of oxygenated blood by rerouting some of it back to the lungs before it could make its way into the general circulatory system via the aorta. She reasoned that an artifically created shunt from one of the nearby arteries to the pulmonary artery might provide an even more efficient means of bypassing the narrowed pulmonary valve (Figure 52). She discussed her idea with Dr. Alfred Blalock, and together they devised the surgical procedure named the *Blalock-Taussig* operation, after its creators.

Few patients with uncorrected tetralogy of Fallot will survive beyond the first or second decades of life. Moreover, their growth is greatly impaired and they are subject to serious, even fatal, complications such as pulmonary hemorrhages, cerebral infarction, and episodes of severe anoxia. For these reasons, surgical treatment is recommended. The procedure of total correction (Figure 52) of tetralogy of Fallot, using the heart-lung machine, is now preferred by most surgeons when the patient reaches the age of five or six and remains in satisfactory condition until this time. However, if a child develops increasing symptoms, a palliative operation, such as the Blalock-Taussig shunting procedure between the subclavian artery and the pulmonary artery; or the Potts procedure of anastomosis between the descending thoracic aorta and the left pulmonary artery; or the Waterston procedure of anastomosis between the ascending aorta and the right pulmonary artery, may be suggested at an earlier age and, occasionally, in infancy. Later, at a second-stage operation, usually performed when the patient is between five and eight years of age, total correction is accomplished. More recently, however, some surgeons are recommending total correction as the initial procedure in all cases, even those requiring operation in infancy.

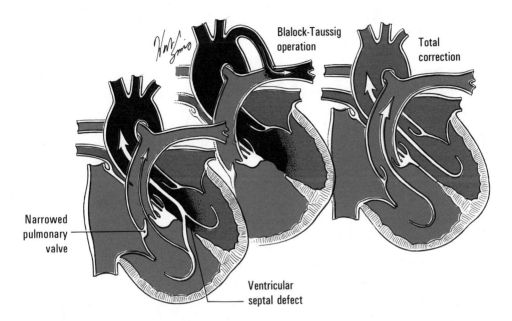

Figure 52. Anatomical abnormalities of heart in tetralogy of Fallot and methods of surgical correction

The results of the operation are excellent. In uncomplicated cases, the risk is less than 3 percent; even in patients requiring operation at an early age, the risk is only about 5 or 6 percent. Studies on patients ten years after complete repair have provided gratifying results, with more than 90 percent alive and well, and leading productive lives.

Defects of the Septum

Defects of the septum, or wall between the right and left chambers of the heart, often referred to as a hole in the heart, are among the most common congenital abnormalities. They may occur in the septum between the two upper chambers of the heart *(atrial septal defects)* or between the two lower chambers *(ventricular septal defects)* (Figure 53).

There are several different kinds of atrial septal defects, the most common being the type in which, despite the size of the hole, there is a remnant of the septum around the defect. In some cases, this remnant may be partially absent, usually on the back side of the heart. Another variation, termed sinus venosus, occurs in the upper part of the septum and is often associated with an abnormal connection of the right superior pulmonary vein which allows blood to flow directly into the right atrium instead of the left atrium. Still another, termed ostium primum, is a partial form of a defect called common atrioventricular canal in which the mitral valve is cleft.

The defect between the two upper chambers of the heart allows blood to flow in either direction. In most cases, however, blood flows from the left atrium into the right, creating what is termed a left-to-right shunt because of the increased pressure on the left side. Depending upon the size of the opening, the shunt may cause a several-fold increase in blood flow to the lungs and thus increase the burden on the heart. Occasionally, because of elevation of pressure in the right atrium due to other complications of the condition or to an increased resistance in the lungs, blood flows from right to left. Indeed, this may take place because of pulmonary vascular changes which cause an initially left-to-right shunt to become reversed. This sometimes is the consequence of allowing a large left-to-right shunt to remain uncorrected.

Most patients with atrial septal defects tolerate the abnormality so well that disabling symptoms do not develop until adulthood. Growth and development are usually normal, although occasional heart failure and retardation of growth occur in infancy. There may be some symptoms of mild fatigability and shortness of breath during periods of exertion, and the heart might be slightly or moderately enlarged.

Surgical correction of the defect is advisable. While it may be necessary to operate at an early age, ideally surgery should be done when the child reaches five or six. However, the operation can give good results even in patients over sixty years of age.

The operation is performed using the heart-lung machine, and correction of the defect may be accomplished by one of several ways, depending upon the type of defect. Some can be closed simply by suturing the edges of the defect together. Others may require a patch of Dacron or pericardium sutured and placed in proper position to close the defect and to divert the pulmonary venous flow into the proper chamber, the left atrium (Figure 53). In other cases, repair of the mitral valve may also be required.

Results of operation are excellent, with virtually no mortality in uncomplicated cases involving children and young adults. Even in older patients the risk of operation is only about 5 percent.

Ventricular septal defects consist of a hole between the two lower chambers of the heart, the right and left ventricles (Figure 53). They are among the most common type of congenital heart disease. The defect varies in position and size but in most cases it produces a left-to-right shunt because of the higher pressure in the left ventricle. This causes a greatly increased blood flow to the lungs and puts a burden on the heart.

The effect of this condition on the patient varies, depending upon its type and size, as well as blood flow through the defect. Spontaneous closure may occur in some patients with small defects and, for this reason, such patients who are without symptoms should be observed over a period of several years. On the other hand, some infants with greatly increased blood flow through large defects may die in the early months of life. Others who survive infancy may develop progressive *pulmonary hypertension* that sometimes becomes so severe that the condition is inoperable.

Surgical correction of a large ventricular septal defect is indicated

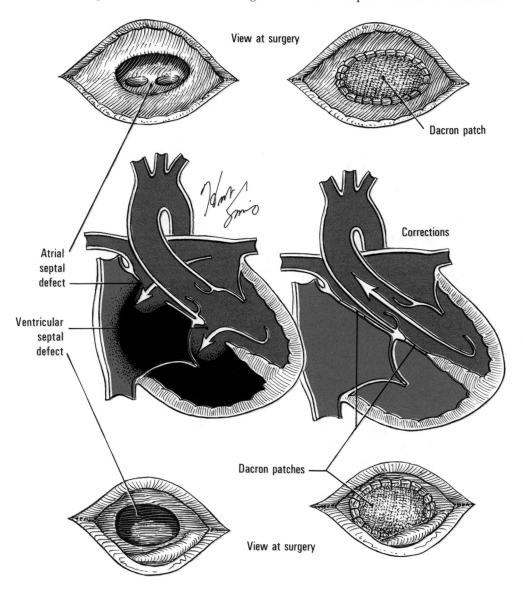

Figure 53. Atrial and ventricular septal defects and their surgical correction

during the first two years of life when there is marked growth retardation, evidence of heart failure or development of progressive pulmonary hypertension. With more moderate-sized defects, the operation may be delayed until the age of four to six years. Children with smaller defects may be observed longer to see if the defect closes without surgery. If the defect persists beyond the age of ten, an operation may be advisable.

Surgical correction of the defect is performed using the heart-lung machine, although some surgeons also use hypothermia. The defect is closed by direct suture closure or by the use of a Dacron patch, depending upon the type and size of the defect (Figure 53). Results of the operation are excellent, with a risk of only about 1 or 2 percent. However, in infants less than six months old and in those with severe pulmonary hypertension, the risk factor increases to about 15 to 20 percent.

Aorticopulmonary Window or Septal Defect

This type of rare congenital abnormality consists of an opening between the ascending aorta and the pulmonary artery (Figure 54). Because pressure is greater in the aorta, blood is shunted from the ascending aorta into the pulmonary artery (a left-to-right shunt) creating an additional burden on the heart and ultimately causing severe pulmonary hypertension. For these reasons, surgery should be done as soon as possible, preferably before the age of two. The operation is performed using the heart-lung machine with closure of the window by means of suture or a patch of Dacron. The risk involved in the operation is relatively small and results are good.

Transposition of the Great Arteries

This is one of the most severe congenital malformations of the heart and the great majority of infants with this defect don't even survive their first year. While it is a rather complex condition with a number of variations, the basic abnormality is the transposition of the aorta and pulmonary artery (Figure 55). Thus, instead of the normal relationship of the aorta to the left ventricle and the pulmonary artery to the right ventricle, the aorta arises from the right ventricle and the pulmonary artery from the left ventricle. Some of these infants survive for a few months, or even for some years, because of the shunting, or mixing, of venous and arterial blood through associated anomalies such as septal defects or patent ductus arteriosus. Most of these infants suffer from cyanosis (as in the blue baby), a blue tinge of the skin resulting from lack of oxygen in the blood, retarded growth and shortness of breath.

Surgical treatment usually is recommended within the first six months to one year of life. Under some circumstances, it may be preferable to perform a *palliative* operation first and postpone the definitive repair for some months or

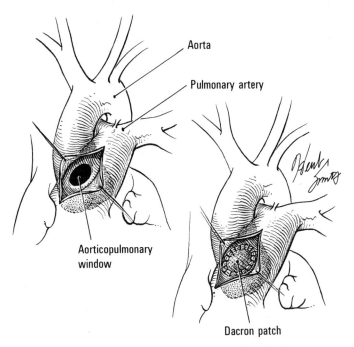

Figure 54. Aorticopulmonary window and surgical correction

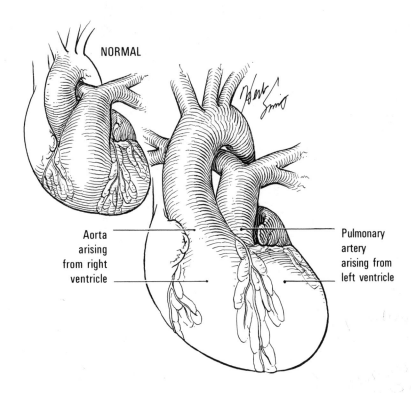

Figure 55. Anatomical abnormalities in transposition of the great arteries

a few years. Several types of definitive procedures for surgical repair have
been devised for this purpose and are designed to restore proper circulation of
arterial and venous blood. Results of the operation are generally good, with a
risk factor ranging from 5 to 30 percent, depending upon the various types of
abnormalities that may be present.

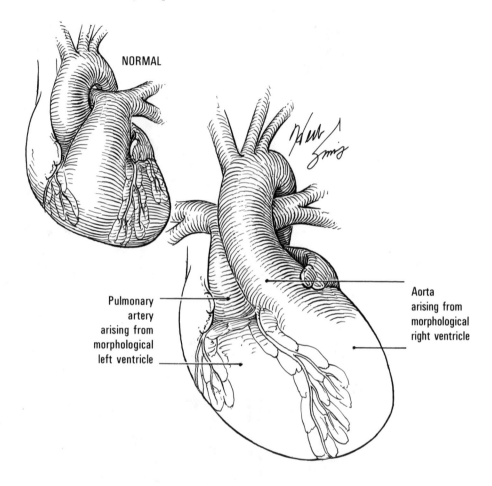

Figure 56. Corrected transposition of the great arteries

There are several different forms and variations of transposition. These
include corrected transposition, a condition in which transposition of the
ventricles accompanies the transposition of the aorta and pulmonary artery
(Figure 56). The normal location of the left ventricle is occupied by a
ventricle that has the morphological (structural) characteristics of the right
ventricle and vice versa. In this situation, the morphological right ventricle
receives blood from the left atrium and pumps it into the aorta. The
morphological left ventricle receives blood from the right atrium and pumps
it into the pulmonary artery. Thus, blood follows a normal pathway through

the heart, hence the term corrected transposition. The presence of associated lesions, such as ventricular septal defects and pulmonic stenosis, determines the prognosis and the need for surgical correction.

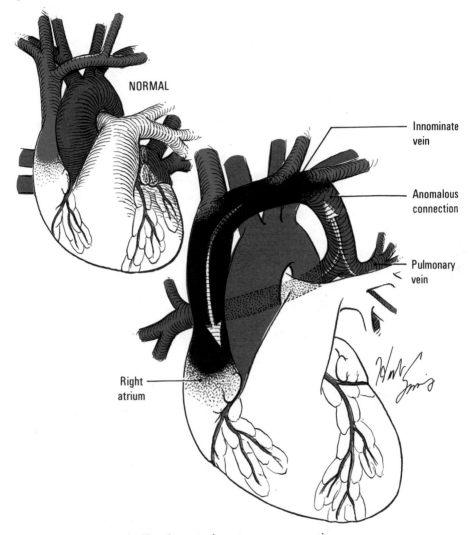

Figure 57. Total anomalous venous connection

Total Anomalous Pulmonary Venous Connection

Normally, the pulmonary veins return oxygenated blood from the lungs to the left atrium of the heart. In the abnormality termed total anomalous venous connection, the pulmonary veins fail to communicate with the left atrium, and instead, discharge their blood into the right atrium by way of one of the major systemic veins (Figure 57). The condition is accompanied by an atrial septal defect or large foramen ovale, allowing the mixed venous and oxygenated blood to be shunted into the left atrium, which permits temporary survival of these infants.

Most infants with this condition develop symptoms shortly after birth: rapid respiration, shortness of breath, feeding difficulties and frequent respiratory infections. If left uncorrected, heart failure and death usually occur within the first year of life. The corrective surgical procedure, with certain variations, is designed to restore the normal return of oxygenated blood from the lungs to the left atrium. Results of the operation are excellent with low risk in patients more than one year of age. In younger infants the risk is somewhat higher.

Aneurysm of the Sinus of Valsalva

This condition is caused by a congenital weakness in the wall of the aorta just above the aortic valves near the origin of the coronary arteries.

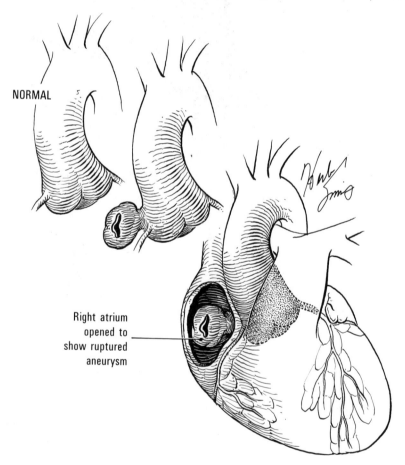

Figure 58. Aneurysm of the sinus of valsalva

This weakness in the wall gradually balloons out to develop a windsock appearance (Figure 58). Symptoms develop only if a rupture occurs, and they vary, depending upon the size of the ruptured opening, from sudden shortness of breath and even rapid heart failure and death, to few or no symptoms.

Surgical treatment is suggested as soon as the diagnosis is made, even in patients who are relatively asymptomatic. Surgical correction of the lesion is performed using the heart-lung machine, and consists of excising the aneurysm and repairing the defect by suture closure or with a Dacron patch. Results of operation are excellent, with an operative risk of less than 5 percent.

Truncus Arteriosus

This form of congenital anomaly is characterized by the absence of direct anatomic continuity between the heart and the pulmonary arterial

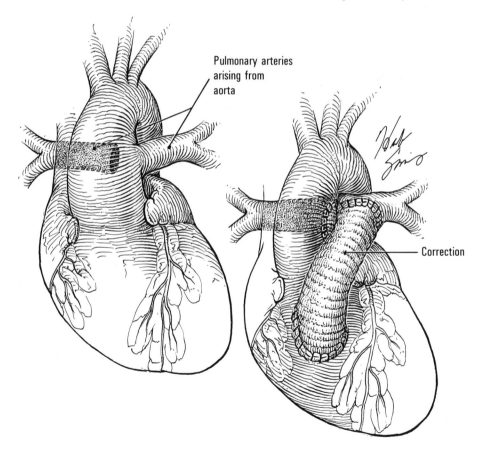

Figure 59. Anatomical abnormality of heart in truncus arteriosus and surgical correction

system. There are several types and variations of this condition. In the most common form, the pulmonary artery arises from the ascending aorta where the pulmonary blood flow originates (Figure 59). A large ventricular septal defect is always present. In another type, there are no identifiable pulmonary arteries, and pulmonary blood flow is by way of the bronchial arteries which arise from the descending aorta to supply blood to the tissues of the lung.

Most infants with this form of congenital heart disease die within the first year of life. A few patients survive beyond this time, but usually develop severe pulmonary vascular disease that renders them inoperable. Until relatively recently, there was no satisfactory surgical procedure for this problem. The surgical procedures that have been developed seem to provide good results. The operation consists of disconnecting the pulmonary artery from the ascending aorta, repairing the defect, closing the ventricular septal defect and connecting the right ventricle to the pulmonary artery by means of an aortic *homograft* or *synthetic graft*. The mortality rate is relatively low— about 12 percent—for children between five and twelve years of age. It is, however, much higher in infants, ranging from 30 to 50 percent.

Congenital Aortic Stenosis

In this type of congenital heart disease there is obstruction to the flow of blood from the left ventricle into the ascending aorta (Figure 60). The blockage may be produced by partial narrowing of the aortic valve itself; by a circumferential ridge of tissue in the ascending aorta just above the valve, termed supravalvular aortic stenosis; or in the outflow tract just below the aortic valve, termed subvalvular aortic stenosis. Still another form of obstruction may be produced by massively *hypertrophied* muscle in the outflow tract of the left ventricle, termed idiopathic hypertrophic subaortic stenosis.

Depending upon the type and severity of the obstruction, infants with this condition may develop acute left ventricular failure and die, or have few symptoms until early childhood when chronic failure may occur. Older children may develop angina, or chest pain, and attacks of weakness or fainting. Sudden death may occur, presumably from ventricular fibrillation. Many patients survive into adult life and then develop increasing obstruction and progressive symptoms.

Surgical treatment is indicated in patients with congenital aortic stenosis who develop symptoms and evidence of left ventricular failure. The procedure is performed using the heart-lung machine. In infants and children particularly, it is usually possible to divide the fused commissures of the stenotic aortic valve. In adults it is often necessary to replace the diseased valve with an artificial valve (for more details, see section on valvular disease in Chapter 13). In supravalvular stenosis, the procedure consists of excision of the ridge of tissue and repair of the opening in the ascending aorta with a patch of Dacron to widen the lumen to normal size. In subvalvular stenosis, the ridge of tissue causing the obstruction is excised. In idiopathic hypertrophic subaortic stenosis, medical treatment is tried first and if symptoms are not controlled adequately, it may be necessary to excise a part of the

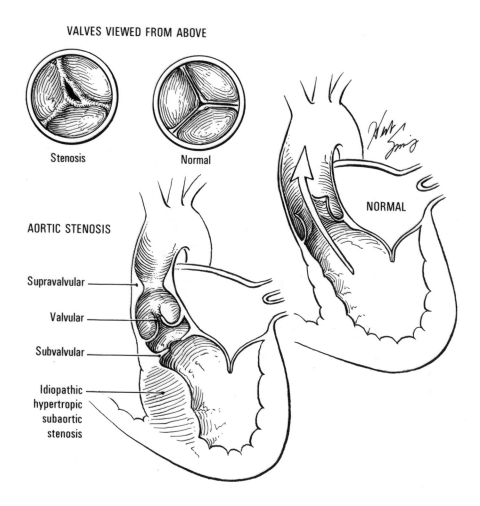

VALVES VIEWED FROM ABOVE

Stenosis

Normal

AORTIC STENOSIS

Supravalvular

Valvular

Subvalvular

Idiopathic hypertropic subaortic stenosis

NORMAL

Figure 60. Types of congenital aortic stenosis

hypertrophied muscle. Results of the operation are generally excellent, with very low risk.

Congenital Mitral Valve Disease

Congenital malformation of the mitral valve may produce narrowing (stenosis) or incompetence of the valve, or a combination of these defects (Figure 61). This condition is often associated with other congenital malformations of the heart such as *endocardial fibroelastosis*, coarctation of the aorta, patent ductus arteriosus and aortic stenosis. Patients with severe malformations are usually gravely ill in infancy and do not survive early

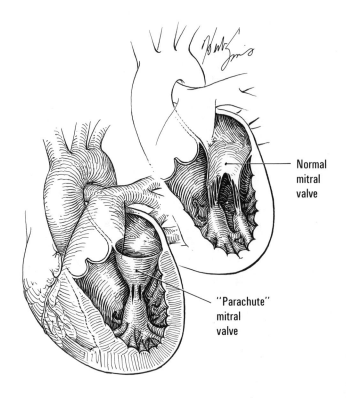

Figure 61. Congenital mitral valve disease

childhood. Patients with milder forms of the disease may reach adulthood. Surgical treatment is directed toward repair of the valve when this is possible, or sometimes replacement of it, and results of surgery are usually good.

Pulmonary Valve Stenosis

This congenital malformation of the pulmonary valve lying between the right ventricle and the pulmonary artery consists of a narrowing of the valve, which produces an added burden on the right ventricle (Figure 62). If there is an associated opening in the atrial septum (a patent foramen ovale or an atrial septal defect), the patient may develop cyanosis. Depending upon the severity of the lesion, patients may die in early infancy or soon thereafter from heart failure. In mild forms of the condition without a septal defect, the patient may have few or no symptoms and tolerate the abnormality quite well.

Surgical treatment should be performed in patients with cyanosis and in those with moderate to severe stenosis. The operation is performed using the heart-lung machine and consists of opening the valve with an incision.

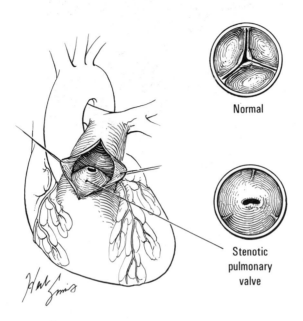

Normal

Stenotic
pulmonary
valve

Figure 62. Pulmonary valve stenosis

Sometimes hypertrophied muscle in the outflow of the right ventricle must be excised. If an atrial septal defect exists, it is closed. Results of the operation are excellent, with virtually no operative risk.

Congenital Tricuspid Atresia

This is a rather grave congenital abnormality. The tricuspid valve is absent; there is a very small right ventricle and an atrial septal defect (Figure 63). There may be some variations in the abnormality. These infants are usually gravely ill and become moderately to markedly cyanotic. Most will die within the first few months of life unless surgery is performed, but this is usually only a palliative treatment rather than definitive correction, and is directed toward increasing pulmonary blood flow. There are several techniques that may be used, including making connections *(anastomoses)* between the superior vena cava and the right pulmonary artery or between the aorta and left pulmonary artery. Results following these operations are good, with relative low risk. There have been some recent efforts to develop a more curative type of operation, but these remain to be properly evaluated.

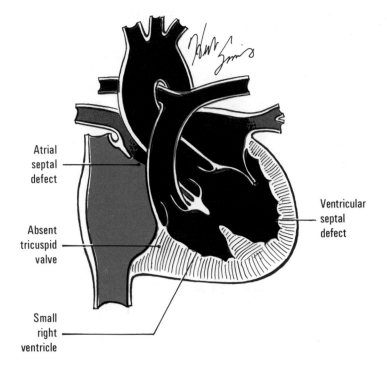

Atrial
septal
defect

Absent
tricuspid
valve

Small
right
ventricle

Ventricular
septal
defect

Figure 63. Congenital tricuspid atresia

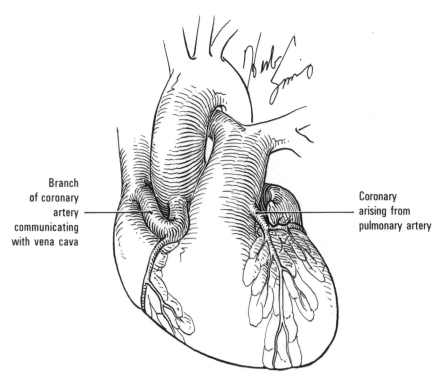

Branch
of coronary
artery
communicating
with vena cava

Coronary
arising from
pulmonary artery

Figure 64. Congenital coronary artery disease

Congenital Coronary Artery Disease

There are two forms of this congenital anomaly of the coronary arteries (Figure 64). In the first type, a large branch of a coronary artery communicates directly with the vena cava, the right atrium, the right ventricle or the pulmonary artery. Blood thus flows from the arterial system directly into the venous system. If this flow is great enough, symptoms will appear and ultimately lead to heart failure. An operation is therefore necessary and consists essentially of closing the anomalous artery by ligation.

The second type is characterized by the left coronary arising from the pulmonary artery. Unless corrected, most of these infants will not survive the first year of life. The operation in this case consists of closing off the artery by ligation or transplanting its origin to the ascending aorta or a systemic artery.

Results following surgery are good in both types of operation.

8

ARTERIOSCLEROSIS
AND
ATHEROSCLEROSIS

M_{OST} cardiovascular catastrophies are caused by an underlying disease called arteriosclerosis or atherosclerosis, the process more commonly known as hardening of the arteries. Arteriosclerosis is a more inclusive term than atherosclerosis and embraces various types of arterial pathology. Professor Jean-Frédéric Lobstein first used the term arteriosclerosis in 1829 to describe several types of arterial disease that affected one or more of the vessel layers. Atherosclerosis is a process that involves predominantly the intimal layer of the artery and most often occurs in medium- to large-sized vessels. The most serious type of atherosclerotic involvement is the *plaque*, which characteristically occurs initially as a focal deposit of lipid within the intimal layer (Figure 65). This lesion, the *atheroma,* is the cause of most heart attacks, strokes and arterial insufficiencies. Ambroise Paré (see Chapter 1) wrote that the early Greeks first used atheroma to refer to a "space containing gruel-like material or porridge."

Very likely, atherosclerosis starts early in life in the United States. Postmortem studies carried out on young soldiers killed in the Korean war

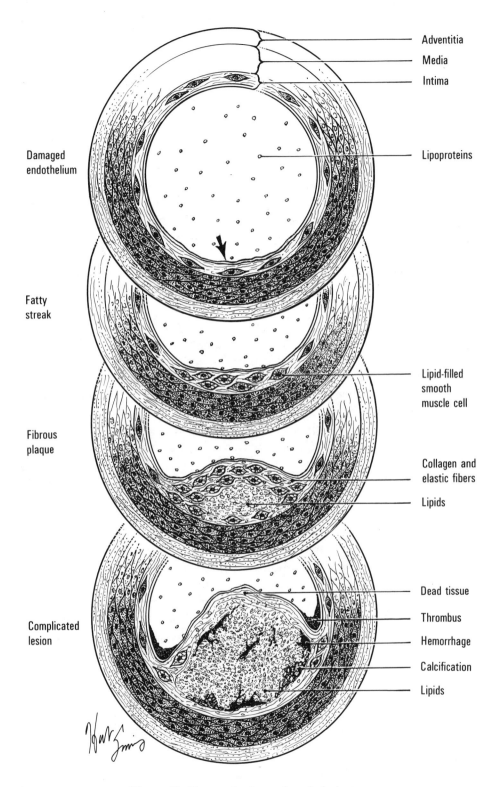

Damaged
endothelium

Fatty
streak

Fibrous
plaque

Complicated
lesion

Adventitia

Media

Intima

Lipoproteins

Lipid-filled
smooth
muscle cell

Collagen and
elastic fibers

Lipids

Dead tissue

Thrombus

Hemorrhage

Calcification

Lipids

Figure 65. Types of atherosclerotic lesions

indicated that many of them had a significant degree of blockage due to atherosclerosis of coronary arteries by the time they were in their mid-twenties.

The intimal layer of the artery is very thin in infancy and thickens as a person gets older. The innermost layer of cells lining the intima and exposed to the bloodstream is called the *endothelium*. Atherosclerosis is believed to begin with damage to this endothelial lining of cells. Just how this occurs is not known. It is possible that elevated blood pressure, high blood cholesterol, stress, or some toxic substance within the blood might contribute to initiating the process. The view that damage to the endothelial layer stimulates the development of atherosclerosis is not new. Rudolph Virchow published a very similar view over one hundred years ago. Once the endothelial cells are damaged, the lipoproteins, the carrier substances in the bloodstream, transport cholesterol and esters of cholesterol into the intima of the artery.

In children and young adults, the thin arterial intima contains very few smooth muscle cells. One hypothesis of how atherosclerosis develops is that cholesterol and its carrier substance from the bloodstream enter the intima through the damaged endothelial lining and stimulate the growth and proliferation of the smooth muscle cells. While the cells of the arterial wall and of other tissues are capable of making cholesterol, it is believed that the bulk of this substance comes from the blood. Most of the cholesterol in normal cells is located within the cell membranes where it helps to regulate the fluidity or stiffness. When too much cholesterol accumulates within the cells and their membranes, a dysfunction results, which could be one of the factors that enhance the abnormal proliferation of smooth muscle cells within the arterial wall. The cell's cholesterol has two sources; some it manufactures itself and some originates in the blood where it is carried in the low-density lipoproteins.

The site where the atherosclerosis occurs is called a *lesion* (Figure 65). One of the earliest changes that can be shown in the development of atherosclerosis is a focal accumulation of cholesterol and its *esters*, which presumably is a consequence of damage to the endothelium. An increase in the quantity of smooth muscle cells, that is, a proliferation of these cells, occurs within the intima. Lipids accumulate within the intima, both inside the proliferating smooth muscle cells and, as a consequence of cell death or necrosis, outside of them. There is a loosening or swelling of the ground substances surrounding the cells of the artery's wall. This change appears to be associated with an increase in complex carbohydrates within the intima. It is believed that smooth muscle cells from the media of the artery migrate into the intima causing further thickening, damage and necrosis. These smooth muscle cells make the extra-cellular substances, collagen and elastic tissue, which may be looked upon as a repair mechanism. These substances accumulate and contribute to the development of the lesion.

Based on their structural appearance, atherosclerotic lesions are usually divided into three categories. One is the fatty streak, which is seen in animals and in all human societies (Figure 65). Fatty streaks begin early in life and, depending on their location, may regress or disappear, stay constant or even progress. The earliest fatty streaks to appear are usually near the aortic outlet from the heart; next are those in the rest of the thoracic aorta; and the last are in the abdominal aorta and coronary arteries. Except in Western societies, fatty streaks do not progress to form more dangerous types of atheromatous lesions. There is much disagreement among pathologists as to whether the individual fatty streak is a precursor of a *fibrous plaque,* or complicated lesion. As mentioned earlier, one of the hallmarks of the development of atherosclerosis is the desposit of cholesterol and its esters in the arterial wall. In the fatty streak, which tends to be a flat lesion, much of the cholesterol and cholesterol esters are inside the cell; that is, they are intracellular. The yellow color of the lesion is attributed to foam cells which are fat-filled smooth muscle cells within the intima. Hence, there is some logic in associating high levels of cholesterol in the blood with an increased tendency to develop atherosclerosis. This presumes that the higher the cholesterol in the bloodstream, the faster it will tend to enter the arterial wall.

A second type of atherosclerotic lesion is called the fibrous plaque (Figure 65). Most of the fats in a fibrous plaque are outside of the cells and they, along with broken-down cells, form a core that is covered by a cap of *collagen tissue,* elastic fibers and smooth muscle cells filled with fat. The cap extends, or protrudes, out into the lumen of the artery. Whereas the fatty streak appears yellow, the fibrous plaque is grayish or whitish in appearance.

The third and most dangerous type of atherosclerotic lesion is called the complicated lesion or plaque. This plaque contains a core of lipid material, mainly cholesterol and cholesterol esters, in a center of dead tissue. Hemorrhage, thrombosis, tissue destruction and calcification may convert a fibrous plaque into a complicated lesion.

A number of theories have been proposed to explain the development of atherosclerosis, but no single one completely and satisfactorily accounts for all of the observations that have been made about this disease. To be valid, any theory about the cause and development of atherosclerosis must be consistent with what is known about its relationship to age, sex, *serum cholesterol,* diet and other risk factors, and its pathological characteristics. Man develops clinically significant atherosclerosis, while other species, including other mammals, do not. The disease is virtually nonexistent in parts of Asia and Africa. In an extensive study, called the International Atherosclerosis Project, carried out by H. C. McGill and J. P. Strong, it was shown that there is much more atherosclerosis in black and white populations in the United States as compared to similar groups in South America and Central America. The incidence of atherosclerosis increases with age; in one report, autopsies showed that approximately 50 percent of the men between the ages of fifty and sixty had significant atherosclerosis, while above the age of seventy, 90 percent were affected. Coronary atherosclerosis affects white males almost twice as frequently as it does women prior to menopause. Such sex differences have not been found in blacks. The atheroma is characterized by the focal deposition of lipids, especially cholesterol and its esters, the composition of which closely parallels that of the serum cholesterol. The atheroma is not only focal, but also tends to occur in arteries at sites of stress. Atherosclerotic lesions may be produced in animals by feeding them a high cholesterol, high saturated-fat diet. In population studies in Western countries, there is a correlation between risk of developing clinically significant artery disease and the level of serum cholesterol. A correlation can also be made between the intake of saturated fat and animal fat and the incidence of coronary atherosclerosis in various societies.

Another theory of atherosclerosis, which proposes that there is a progressive degeneration of the arterial wall with age, does not account for sex differences in the disease, the distribution of the disease in various societies and the occurrence of severe disease in many young people. A theory involving trauma postulates that at points of stress in the artery or when there is a chronic increase in blood pressure, the endothelium may be damaged and its permeability to lipids increased. Mechanical trauma is very likely one factor that predisposes certain parts of the vascular tree to develop atherosclerosis, but it cannot explain the whole picture.

One of the characteristics of atherosclerosis is that it is a focal disease. The focal and patchy distribution of lesions was emphasized by William Councilman, who used the term nodular arteriosclerosis to describe this phenomenon. The focal nature of atherosclerosis is indeed one of its puzzles and perhaps one of the clues to understanding what causes it and how to prevent it. Some studies have suggested that local stress contributes to the development of a lesion at a particular site within the artery.

John B. Duguid has reintroduced the thrombogenic theory originally proposed by Baron Karl von Rokitansky in 1852. This theory proposes that the atherosclerotic plaque within the intima occurs because of the formation of small multiple blood clots which are eventually converted into scar tissue. However, the formation of such thrombi within the intima more likely is because of secondary rather than primary changes in the evolution of the atheromatous plaque. Another related theory is that intimal thickening occurs because of repeated hemorrhaging within the intima. As a consequence of recurrent hemorrhage, it is suggested that abnormal vascular patterns develop within the intima. The theories of intramural hemorrhage and of thrombogenesis account for only a small part of the overall picture, since neither explains the relationship between hypercholesterolemia and atherosclerosis.

Dr. Earl Benditt of Seattle has made the very interesting observation that an atherosclerotic lesion seems to be derived from a single cell type.

Doctor Benditt and his co-workers found that the proportion of cells undergoing division is about ten times higher in the blood vessels of rats whose blood pressure is raised as compared with normal rats. They speculate that there may be viruses or other toxic agents that cause transformation of a sensitive cell within the arterial wall to initiate the development of a lesion. This transformation might be similar to that which occurs when a cancer or neoplasm develops.

Other researchers have shown that the growth and proliferation of smooth muscle cells from the arterial wall can be stimulated by exposure to a variety of substances like *hyperlipidemic serum,* low density lipoproteins and blood platelets, which are involved in blood clotting.

To sum up, the most crucial steps in the evolution of an atherosclerotic lesion are 1) damage to the endothelial lining, 2) the focal accumulation of intimal lipids, 3) the proliferation of the smooth muscle cells of the arterial wall, 4) cell death and injury and 5) the formation of a necrotic, lipid-rich core. The precise interrelationships and causes of these effects are not known. Cholesterol and low-density lipoproteins accumulate and may influence several of these phenomena. Collagen, elastic fibers and ground substances accumulate as secondary effects.

How does the intimal plaque affect the rest of the arterial wall? As you recall from Chapter 5, the adventitia of the artery contains connective tissue and small blood vessels, the vasa vasorum, which supply oxygen to the outer half of the arterial media. The inner half of the media, on the other hand, obtains its oxygen supply by diffusion of oxygen from the bloodstream. When a plaque develops, the blood and oxygen supply from the vasa vasorum and the bloodstream may become inadequate because of the thickening of the wall, which may lead to further damage of the artery. Bleeding may occur into a plaque and the wall may become sufficiently damaged at the site of the plaque so that a blood clot or thrombosis forms. What happens to an atherosclerotic plaque once it forms determines the clinical complications for the individual. If the plaque develops to the point that it protrudes into the lumen or opening of the artery, it may produce symptoms such as cramps or pain in the legs during walking, chest pain during physical or emotional exertion, and dizziness. These symptoms, which result from the impairment of blood flow, vary, depending upon which particular vascular bed is affected.

An important consideration in this disease process is the development of collateral circulation, nature's method of compensating for the obstruction of blood flow. Small arteries arising from branches above the obstruction develop connections to small arteries communicating with arteries below the obstruction (Figure 66). In this way, some blood flows around the obstructed segment to provide circulation to the arterial bed below the blockage. Although the circulation provided by this compensatory mechanism may be adequate to maintain viability and some function, it is not usually enough to permit normal function. The adequacy of the collateral channels varies from individual to individual.

A common misconception concerning atherosclerosis is that the disease is a single entity. Nothing could be further from the truth. In fact, there are a number of different patterns of atherosclerosis, and failure to understand this concept could lead to inappropriate therapy and expectations. One pattern involves the distribution of the lesions (Figure 67). In some individuals, the disease may be confined to the peripheral arteries and the coronary arteries,

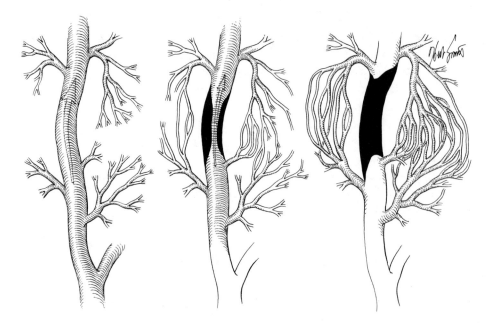

Figure 66. The development of collateral circulation may compensate for the obstruction to blood flow caused by atherosclerotic occlusive disease.

with the aorta and the cerebral arteries completely free of the disease. Other patients have atherosclerosis limited to the coronary vessels, while in some only the arterial supply to the central nervous system is affected. There are patients who have the disease limited to the aorta, to the visceral arteries or to the arteries carrying blood to the kidneys. Many patients have more than one area affected. Generally, the coronary arteries tend to be affected earlier in life; the mean age for heart attacks is lower than for strokes or peripheral arterial disease.

A second pattern relates to the rate of progression of the disease. In some patients it is extremely rapid, leading to death within less than a year after the initial onset of symptoms. This pattern is sometimes called "galloping atherosclerosis." Other patients show manifestations of atherosclerosis in one vascular bed and have no further progression even after many years. We have seen patients at The Methodist Hospital in Houston who were operated on to remove an isolated plaque over twenty years ago. After two decades of close follow-up and scrutiny, some of these people showed absolutely no further

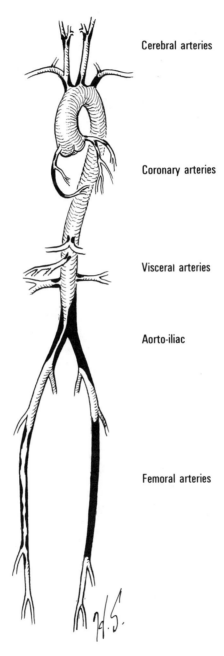

Cerebral arteries

Coronary arteries

Visceral arteries

Aorto-iliac

Femoral arteries

Figure 67. Anatomic patterns of atherosclerotic occlusive disease

signs of atherosclerosis. Unfortunately, such individuals are the exception rather than the rule. In most cases, there is some degreee of progression over a period of years.

A third pattern of atherosclerosis relates to the characteristics of the lesion. We have referred to the atherosclerotic, or complicated, plaque which usually leads to occlusive disease. Instead of an occlusion, some patients develop a ballooning-out of the artery, called an aneurysm, which will be discussed in detail in Chapter 12. While we do not know the risk factors and biochemical influences which lead to the various types of atherosclerosis, we believe that knowledge about these patterns and the factors that contribute to them may lead to an understanding of the susceptibility of the individual to the development of the ailment. This is one of the most fundamental and unanswered questions in the entire cardiovascular field.

9

CORONARY ARTERY DISEASE

*W*E have already referred to the fact that cardiovascular disease represents the major cause of death in our society. Each year in the United States alone, approximately one million people die from various forms of cardiovascular disease; about 600,000 to 700,000 die from heart attacks or coronary artery disease. Finland and the United States lead all other countries in the death rate from coronary artery disease. Since the beginning of the twentieth century, there has been a tremendous increase in the recorded death rate from heart attacks in the Western world. The explanation for this increase is not known. Part of the apparent increase may be due to the significant decrease in deaths resulting from other causes, especially infection. Physicians also have become more aware of cardiovascular disease and can diagnose it more accurately. However, as discussed in Chapter 1, we believe that there has been an actual increase in the incidence of coronary artery disease in Western societies.

Various theories have been proposed, such as an increase in the consumption of animal fat, cigarette smoking, and the consumption of sugar, as well as a decrease in exercise, the growth of industrialization and an increase in the day to day pressures and stresses to which individuals are subjected.

In the chapter on preventive maintenance, the various risk factors for cardiovascular disease and, in particular, for coronary disease, are discussed and suggestions are made about ways to try to diminish the risk. The major risk factors for premature coronary disease are generally considered to be an elevation of serum cholesterol, elevation of blood pressure or hypertension, and cigarette smoking. Unfortunately, there is no current scientific evidence to prove absolutely that correction of an abnormal risk factor will necessarily protect an individual against the likelihood of having an early heart attack. Several studies are now being carried out by the National Heart, Lung and Blood Institute to determine whether or not reduction of blood pressure, cigarette smoking and serum cholesterol will protect individuals who have these risk factors but are free of manifestations of cardiovascular disease.

In the recently completed Coronary Drug Project, men who already had one or more heart attacks were treated with one of four medications: estrogen, or female sex hormone; dextrothyroxine, an analog of the normal thyroid hormone; clofibrate, a drug that reduces primarily an elevation of blood triglyceride but to a much lesser extent also cholesterol; and niacin, or nicotinic acid, a B vitamin which lowers both cholesterol and triglyceride. For each group of participants that received a medication, there was a control group who received a placebo, or fake medication, which was the equivalent of a sugar pill. None of the groups receiving any of the medication had any reduction in total mortality or in the death rate from heart attacks. In fact, patients receiving two of the drugs, estrogen and dextrothyroxine, had a higher rate of complications than patients in the control group. These medications were discontinued as soon as the adverse effects were discovered. Clofibrate gave no protection against death from heart attacks or cardiovascular disease, and its use was associated with complications such as an increase in the occurrence of gall stones and an increase in the tendency to form blood clots. Niacin did not decrease the mortality rate but did reduce the incidence of nonfatal heart attacks. What can be learned from this study is that more powerful medications to lower cholesterol are needed and that it is important to detect people who are at risk before they develop heart attacks. However, the other nationwide studies referred to earlier will have to be completed before a definitive statement can be made as to whether or not practical measures that are currently available to correct the risk factors will protect the individual from the ravages of coronary heart disease and its complications.

There is some hope from preliminary data which suggest that the death rate from coronary artery disease in the United States may have reached a peak and may have actually declined over the past ten years. Unfortunately, at the present state of knowledge, it is not possible to identify which changes occurred over the past ten years to account for this apparent decline.

Because of the importance of coronary artery disease, a somewhat detailed discussion of this problem is appropriate. Despite the relatively small size of the heart, about 20 percent of the total blood flow is needed to provide nourishment for the heart itself. There are two vessels called the coronary

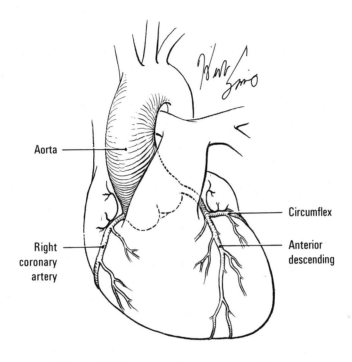

Figure 68. The normal coronary arteries

arteries which originate from the ascending aorta shortly after it leaves the heart (Figure 68). They have been named the coronary arteries because they encircle the heart like a crown. About one inch from its origin, the left coronary splits into two vessels, one called the *left anterior descending* and the other the *circumflex*. These designations indicate the routes these arteries take along the heart. The circumflex follows a curving groove along the wall that separates the left atrium from the left ventricle. The left anterior descending artery runs along the groove on the front of the heart between the left and right ventricles. The right coronary artery curves to the right between the right atrium and the right ventricle to reach the groove between the two ventricles on the back of the heart. A fine network of vessels arises from these arteries and serves as tributaries to feed the heart.

In an adult, a coronary artery measured from beginning to end is only four or five inches long. The lumen or bore of the artery is about one-eighth of an inch in diameter. Approximately fifteen gallons of blood are pumped through these arteries each hour. A reduction in the lumen by over 60 to 70 percent usually is required before clinical symptoms of reduced blood flow will appear.

The major cause of coronary artery obstruction is the development of atherosclerotic plaques. Characteristically, plaques are found in the first three centimeters of the anterior descending branch of the left coronary artery. The right coronary artery is most frequently affected in its first five centimeters, and the circumflex artery just beyond its splitting off from the main trunk. When the lumen is so obstructed that an inadequate amount of blood and oxygen is available to support the needs of the heart muscle, we refer to the condition as myocardial ischemia. When this sequence of events occurs, it usually results in a form of chest discomfort that is called *angina pectoris* and that is brought on by physical and emotional exertion. The attack may begin with a choking sensation or feeling of weight pushing against the breastbone. The most frequent location for the discomfort is beneath the sternum, or breastbone. The sensation may extend up into the neck and down the arm, particularly along the small finger side of the left arm. In describing angina pectoris, the patient often will symbolize the discomfort by squeezing his fist. The pain usually is not sharp or superficial, but is deep and squeezing and aching in character.

In fact, the patient may actually deny that he has "pain." Typically, the attack is brought on by exertion, either physical or emotional, and is relieved by rest. It almost always lasts longer than one minute, but generally less than ten. Taking nitroglycerin under the tongue usually gives relief of an attack within one to three minutes. The symptoms usually subside more quickly when the person is in a sitting or standing position. When lying down, the ventricular filling is increased, which raises cardiac output but also increases myocardial oxygen consumption, which may account for the exacerbation of the anginal symptoms in this position. The Roman philosopher and author Seneca probably provided the first recorded description of angina pectoris when he wrote over nineteen hundred years ago that "the attack is very short and like a storm. It usually ends within an hour. I have undergone all bodily informaties; but none appear to be more grievous." The British physician William Heberden observed angina pectoris in 1768 and described it in a classic report as follows, "They who are affected with it are seized while they are walking (more especially if it be uphill, and soon after eating) with a painful and most disagreeable sensation in the breast but seems as if it could extinguish life if it were to increase or continue; but the moment they stand still all this uneasiness vanishes."

The great British anatomist Dr. John Hunter added a painful auto-biographical note of understanding about angina pectoris. This violent-tempered man recognized that he himself suffered from angina and that painful attacks were brought on by emotional upheaval. He prophesized his fear that his behavior would one day bring about his death, due to constant quarreling with his colleagues at the London Hospital. After a particularly bitter dispute one day, Dr. Hunter left a board meeting, and in the words of Sir William Osler, "In silent rage and in the next room gave a deep groan

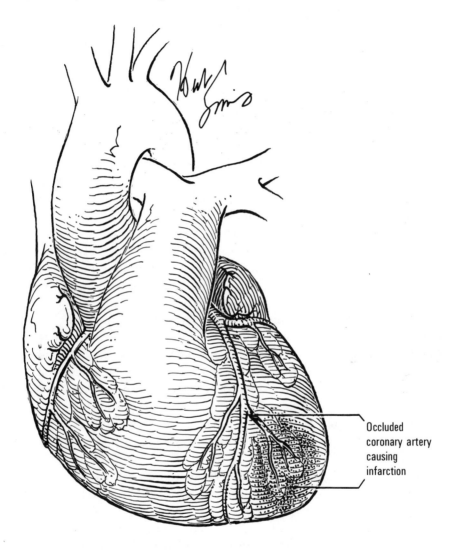

Figure 69. Myocardial infarction caused by blockage of a branch of the anterior descending coronary artery

and fell down dead." It remained for William Jenner, near the end of the eighteenth century, armed with the understanding of the circulatory system provided by William Harvey, to make the connection between angina pectoris and the coronary arteries. To sum up, substernal chest pain of a squeezing or aching quality, brought on by exercise, relieved within a few minutes by rest, and lasting more than one minute but less than ten minutes has about a 95 percent likelihood of being angina pectoris.

Patients with atherosclerotic disease of the coronary arteries are subject to myocardial ischemia or lack of oxygen to the heart muscle. If this results from a sudden or acute occlusion of a coronary artery, the patient will suffer a heart attack. The medical term used to designate the heart attack is a myocardial infarction, or coronary thrombosis (Figure 69). The term myocardial infarction means death of cells of tissues of the heart. These are acute electrocardiographic changes that are diagnosic of a myocardial infarction and which appear within minutes to hours of the critical onset. Subsequently, the electrocardiogram shows abnormalities which evolve over days to months (Figure 70). In the majority of cases, if the coronary arteries are examined after an individual dies of a myocardial infarction, a blood clot will be found in one or more of the coronary arteries. The longer the patient survives after the onset of symptoms, the greater the liklihood of finding a clot in an artery. Pathologists and cardiologists do not agree among themselves which is the cart and which is the horse as far as thrombosis and myocardial infarction are concerned. Some think that a thrombus, or blood clot, is formed in an artery, shutting off the blood supply, and leading to a myocardial infarction. Others believe that the infarction is the cause of the thrombosis, rather than the effect of it. At any rate, the two phenomena are related and the net effect is to cut off the blood and oxygen supply, which causes ischemia in an area of the heart and death of the heart muscle. Coronary atherosclerosis, coronary occlusion and myocardial ischemia and infarction are closely related phenomena but do not always show a one-to-one relationship. Some patients with severe atherosclerosis exhibit only minimal symptoms and evidence of ischemia. In fact, patients may have totally occluded coronary arteries and in some instances remain asymptomatic with a relatively normally functioning myocardium. The development of collateral paths of circulation probably plays a highly important role in such patients.

The area of an infarction may be small or diffuse. If the full thickness of the myocardium is involved, from the endocardial surface to the epicardium, the infarction is termed transmural. The most frequent site of acute occlusion is the anterior descending branch of the left coronary artery. This often results in infarction of the anterior segment of the interventricular septum, the apex and front third of the lateral wall of the left ventricle. Occlusion of the right coronary artery ranks second in frequency. This vessel supplies the back or posterior part of the left ventricle. Occlusion of the circumflex artery affects the lateral wall of the left ventricle.

Anywhere from 15 to 25 percent of patients who have a myocardial infarction die, and it is distressing that over one-half of these deaths occur before the victim can reach the hospital. One cause of death, and the most important one in patients who never get to the hospital alive, is an irregular heart rhythm, or cardiac arrhythmia. As discussed earlier, the heart has its own electrical conduction system. If the area of damage from the infarction affects the conduction tissue of the heart, an irregularity may result and may progress to a condition called ventricular fibrillation. This results in an electrical form of death similar to that occurring in electrocution: the heart

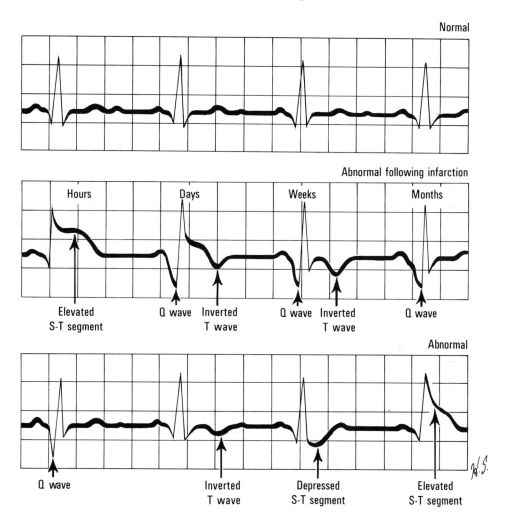

Figure 70. Comparison of a normal electrocardiogram with the various abnormalities that may occur with coronary artery disease

beats rapidly but ineffectively and blood is not pumped out to supply the body. The brain cannot survive more than four to six minutes without blood and oxygen. Another cause of death in connection with a myocardial infarction is heart failure. This phenomenon is directly related to the size of the infarction, that is, to the amount of myocardial tissue that is destroyed. If the amount of dead tissue is so great that the heart can no longer effectively pump blood to the tissues, then blood will collect in the lungs and the patient may die of heart failure. If the subendocardial muscle is involved in the infarction, a blood clot, or thrombus, may form on the subendocardial surface. Such a clot is called a *mural thrombus*. After healing of the heart muscle, a part of the mural thrombus may break off to be carried as an embolus to another tissue. Emboli can be very dangerous if they are carried to a kidney or the brain, often causing a stroke in the latter case. A lethal complication of a myocardial infarction is rupture of the myocardium. This may occur if the wall of the heart becomes so soft and weakened that it perforates with the stress of contracting. This is a catastrophic situation in which blood rapidly fills the chamber around the heart, interferes with filling of the heart and death results. This phenomenon is called *cardiac tamponade*. Other complications of heart attacks include rupture of the interventricular septum and development of insufficiency of the mitral valve due to damage of the papillary muscle or chordae tendinae. These conditions may necessitate surgical intervention. Ten to twenty-one days after the heart attack, the patient may have a recurrence of chest pain due to what is called a postmyocardial syndrome. In this condition the patient has not experienced another myocardial infarction but instead has an inflammatory condition characterized by evidence of pericarditis and pneumonitis, or inflammation of the lungs. A long-term complication is the formation of an aneurysm involving the wall of the heart, due to its weakening. Such an aneurysm may interfere with cardiac function to the extent that it may eventually require surgical removal.

The Diagnosis of Coronary Artery Disease

In the evaluation of a patient with chest pain, the physician gets much more useful information from the patient's history than from the physical examination. There are a number of possibilities that the physician must keep in mind. One is that the chest pain does not originate from the heart and that the patient does not have coronary artery disease. At the other end of the spectrum is the situation in which the chest pain is angina pectoris and the patient does have coronary artery disease. The fact that a patient has chest pain and coronary artery disease does *not* necessarily prove that the pain is coming from the coronary arteries. Many patients have significant blockage of the coronary arteries for years without experiencing clinical symptoms. Thus, such a patient could have coronary artery disease which was asymptomatic and might have chest pain that was noncardiac in origin. Another possibility is the patient with typical or atypical angina pectoris but with no blockage of the coronary arteries. In such patients the pain is thought to be due to spasm of the coronary arteries or to "small vessel" disease in the minute distal branches of the coronary arteries.

The resting electrocardiogram is not a sensitive indicator of coronary artery disease. If the patient has had a prior myocardial infarction, Q waves may be present (Figure 70). However, Q waves may be produced by other conditions. Inversion of T waves and depression of ST segments may be seen on the electrocardiogram of some patients with coronary artery disease, but these are relatively nonspecific findings. In one variant pattern of angina, called Printzmetal's angina, there is marked ST segment elevation during the anginal attack but the electrocardiogram later reverts to normal. ST elevation also is present during an acute myocardial infarction and may persist in patients who develop a ventricular aneurysm.

The best *noninvasive* test for coronary artery disease today is the exercise electrocardiogram. This is an outgrowth of the "Master's test," developed a number of years ago by Dr. Arthur Master of New York City. As currently performed, the test uses either a treadmill or a bicycle for the patient to exercise on. Changes in the electrocardiogram during and after exercise are recorded. One important piece of information, of course, is whether the patient actually experiences chest pain during the exercise procedure, which is aimed at achieving a certain targeted heart rate. It is important to see whether a cardiac irregularity, or arrhythmia, occurs during the test. Many patients have relatively minor arrhythmias which tend to disappear with exercise. If, on the other hand, the irregularity becomes worse or if the patient develops a life-threatening arrhythmia during exercise, this is essential to know in regulating the kind and degree of physical activity the patient can perform. The most commonly used information from an exercise electrocardiogram is the extent of ST segment depression below the resting or baseline value. When the established level of ST depression is exceeded, usually 1 to 1.5 millimeters below the baseline, the test is said to be positive and the result, or response, is described as *ischemic.* This simply implies that a segment of the myocardium is receiving an insufficient supply of blood and oxygen during exercise. Many patients who have already had a myocardial infarction and who have Q waves on the resting electrocardiogram, do not show an ischemic response with exercise. This result presumably implies that the remaining amount of myocardial tissue does receive adequate blood and oxygen during exercise. The test has the highest likelihood of accurately predicting coronary artery disease when it is applied in a group of patients who have a high incidence of this disease. When applied to a large group of asymptomatic individuals who have a low incidence of coronary artery disease, the likelihood of having a false positive test is greatly increased. Therefore, the main use of the exercise cardiogram is in the clinical evaluation of the patient with chest pain that is suspected to represent angina pectoris.

There are other noninvasive tests available to the physician for evaluation of the heart, but they are not usually of great value in determining the presence and/or extent of coronary artery narrowing. The physician usually cannot learn very much from an ordinary chest x-ray. Fluoroscopic study of the heart may show calcification of the coronary arteries, which in patients under age fifty-five has a high correlation with some degree of coronary obstruction.

Another noninvasive test is echocardiography, or the use of sound waves to study the heart's movements. This procedure allows visualization of the posterior wall of the left ventricle and of the ventricular septum. Echocardiography is useful in diagnosing cardiac diseases which may mimic the chest pain of coronary artery disease, but it is of relatively limited value in diagnosing coronary artery disease.

There is another group of tests that may be referred to as myocardial imaging, or blood pool imaging, which involves the use of radionuclides to provide valuable information about the state of the myocardium. One such test produces an image of the myocardium and detects impaired perfusion of the myocardium by the coronary arteries. This provides information that can be correlated with the anatomic obstruction shown by coronary arteriography, to be discussed later. A second type of radionuclide test produces an image of the blood pools within the ventricles and can be used to assess the contractility of specific regions of the ventricle, as well as the ventricle as a whole. A third type of test actually can detect and outline the area of a myocardial infarction.

At the present state of the art, the coronary *arteriogram* provides the most specific and definitive information about the anatomic site and extent of coronary obstruction. Coronary arteriography is performed by inserting a catheter through the brachial or femoral artery and threading it into the ascending aorta to the origin of a coronary artery. A radiopaque dye then is injected to make the coronary artery visible on x-ray movies (Figure 71). After both coronary arteries are injected, the catheter may be threaded through the aortic valve into the left ventricle and more dye is injected in order to view the function of the ventricle, a technique known as ventriculography. This procedure can identify areas of weakness in the wall of the left ventricle, including possible aneurysm formation. At the same time, the catheter is used to take pressure measurements which provide information on the function of the left ventricle.

Coronary vessels as small as one-half of a millimeter in diameter may be seen on the coronary arteriogram. Knowledge of the site and extent of obstruction and of the number of coronary arteries involved enables the physician to evaluate the patient's prognosis and decide upon the best treatment. In general, the less extensive the disease and the fewer vessels involved at the time the disease is discovered, the less rapid will be the further progress of the coronary obstruction. There are some risks involved in coronary arteriography but the death rate per study is far less than one thousandth in the hands of an experienced angiographer.

It is important to keep in mind that while coronary arteriography

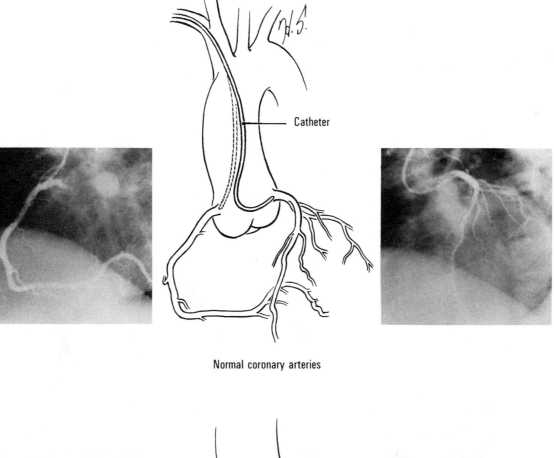

Catheter

Normal coronary arteries

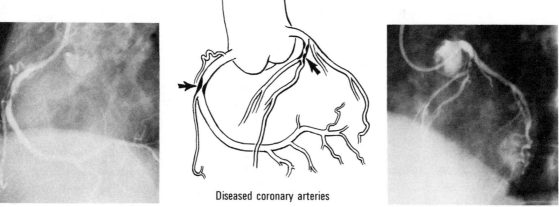

Diseased coronary arteries

Figure 71. Coronary arteriography is performed by taking an x-ray while a radiopaque dye is injected into the coronary arteries. This procedure provides precise information about the anatomic site and extent of coronary artery disease. Normal coronary arteriograms are shown above. Lower coronary arteriograms reveal site of atherosclerotic occlusive disease (arrows).

defines anatomic lesions, it does not identify areas of myocardia ischemia or oxygen insufficiency, and it fails to show "small vessel disease" of the heart. During the coronary arteriography, the dye injected into the left ventricle allows segmental abnormalities of contraction to be visualized. In some instances administration of nitroglycerin will correct the abnormal contractility in a particular segment or region of the myocardium.

The Treatment of Coronary Artery Disease and Its Complications

The more advanced the coronary artery disease, the less likely risk factor intervention will be of value. The time to begin treatment is before any symptoms of the coronary atherosclerosis become apparent, and ideally, prior to the development of a significant degree of atherosclerosis. Usually, the first clinical symptom of coronary artery disease is angina pectoris. The occurence of this symptom means that the oxygen requirements of the myocardium are greater than the coronary arteries can deliver. The rationale for the treatment of this condition, therefore, is to decrease the myocardial oxygen requirements, to increase coronary blood flow, or both.

It should be kept in mind that once a patient develops clinically symptomatic coronary artery disease, sudden death is a possibility. This is caused by an irregularity of the heart rhythm resulting in ventricular fibrillation. Sudden death may also occur independent of myocardial infarction. In this case, the patient dies suddenly and no thrombosis or evidence of infarction is found. Unfortunately, unless the arrhythmia occurs in a place where cardiopulmonary resuscitation can be provided immediately, there is little hope of survival.

Another complication of coronary artery disease is the failure of the heart as a pump. This complication was discussed in conjunction with myocardial infarction. However, some patients develop coronary artery disease and progress to heart failure without evidence of a myocardial infarction.

The drug that has been used the longest for treatment of angina pectoris is nitroglycerin, which usually relieves an anginal attack within one to three minutes and, if taken before a stressful event, may prevent an attack. Despite its long use, we still do not know the precise workings of nitroglycerin, except that it is a vasodilator, and causes relaxation of the smooth muscle tissue in blood vessels. This is probably not its primary effect in relieving angina. More likely the nitroglycerin causes a redistribution of blood flow within the myocardium so that deprived areas receive a more adequate flow, and it causes a decrease in the requirement of the myocardium for oxygen by decreasing tension in the myocardial fibers. The net effect is to improve the relationship between the delivery of oxygen and the work requirement of the myocardium. Medications such as nitroglycerin tend to decrease the oxygen requirements of areas of the myocardium where circulation is deficient. This is another way of saying that the oxygen supply in relation to the work demand of the myocardium is improved.

There are longer-acting drugs than nitroglycerin, which are now available. However, there is little convincing evidence that such agents are any more effective than nitroglycerin.

More recently, the drug *propanolol* has been used to control angina pectoris. This agent decreases the increased oxygen requirements of the heart that the adrenal hormones bring about. But there are limitations to its use. It should not be administered to patients with heart failure or bronchial asthma, and the drug should not be withdrawn suddenly from patients receiving it because a tendency for the aggregation of blood platelets may sharply increase.

One of the most important things that can be done to protect against sudden death is to be aware of the symptoms of myocardial infarction. Sustained chest pain, unrelieved by rest or nitroglycerin after fifteen or twenty minutes, is sufficient cause to seek emergency medical attention. If the chest pain has never been experienced before, attention should be sought upon its onset. The overall mortality for myocardial infarctions is about 15 to 25 percent. One of the reasons for the decrease in mortality from heart attacks in the past ten to fifteen years is because of the development of the ability to monitor patients with real or suspected myocardial infarctions in a coronary care unit. Under these circumstances, if a serious cardiac arrhythmia occurs, it can be corrected quickly by the use of medication or, if necessary, by electric shock. It is astounding that over one-half of the people who die of myocardial infarction die before they reach a hospital. If you cannot reach your physician and you are having chest pains that you think may be caused by a heart attack, do not wait for him to return your call or for his answering service to track him down. Call an ambulance or otherwise go as quickly as possible to the emergency room of the nearest hospital with a coronary care unit.

There has been a dispute for many years concerning the usefulness of anticoagulants in preventing heart attacks. There is very little convincing evidence that the use of these agents will prevent heart attacks. However, there is evidence to suggest that it may be advantageous to anticoagulate patients with heparin at the time of an acute myocardial infarction in order to decrease the likelihood of the formation of a venous blood clot, which could break off and be carried to the lungs to cause a pulmonary embolus. Such treatment is a temporary measure and the anticoagulant is discontinued after the patient is discharged from the hospital.

One area of active research is now directed toward reduction of the size of a myocardial infarction, one of the major factors that determines the disability and death that result from a heart attack. This approach requires intervention soon after the onset of symptoms. During the early phases of an infarction there are areas of the myocardium with a decreased blood supply and diminished oxygen; that is to say, they are hypoxic. *Hypoxia* may lead to a larger area of infarct, to the failure of the heart as a pump or to the occurrence of a fatal arrhythmia. Yet hypoxic areas of the heart potentially may be saved either by improving their metabolic status or by decreasing the amount of work that they have to do. Because the intracellular oxygen level falls, aerobic metabolism diminishes, and an anerobic process (called glycolysis) supersedes, the level of ATP falls, the pH decreases and the cells develop an acidosis. Noradrenalin and adrenalin stores within the myocardium are released. Secretion of these hormones into the circulation from the adrenal gland is the major determinant of the body's metabolic response to the heart attack. Adrenalin causes release of glucose from the liver and noradrenaline stimulates the breakdown of triglyceride fats in adipose tissue to release the fatty acids into the circulation.

The rise in blood sugar and free fatty acids increases the supply of available metabolic substrates to the myocardium. However, these adrenal hormones also result in potentially adverse effects on the myocardium by increasing the peripheral resistance against which the heart must pump, raising the tension of the myocardium and by elevating the contractile state of the heart muscle. There is some evidence, although not considered conclusive at this time, that elevated levels of plasma-free fatty acids may increase the likelihood of serious cardiac arrhythmias.

One approach aimed at improving the metabolic status of the myocardium is the administration of a solution of glucose, insulin and potassium as suggested by Dr. Demitrio Sodi-Pallares. This method aims at increasing the concentration of glucose in the injured heart cell. Administration of glucagon or of potassium, magnesium and apartic acid may have a similar action. Dr. Michael Francis Oliver has suggested the use of agents such as analogs of nicotinic acid to reduce the release of free fatty acids from adipose tissue as a possible means of preventing arrhythmias. Other methods of treatment, aimed at reducing myocardial work requirements, include medications which either lessen the oxygen consumption of the heart or lower blood pressure.

While preliminary results from some of these approaches aimed at reducing the size of infarcts is encouraging, it should be cautioned that physiologic and biochemical measurements of improved perfusion or metabolism must be translated into demonstrable clinical benefits. The approaches just mentioned are still in an experimental stage, but it is hoped that such studies will provide information that will lead to methods by which the mortality and disability from heart attacks will be lowered significantly.

There was a time when patients with myocardial infarctions were kept in bed for long periods of time. This is no longer true. As already discussed, the great majority of patients recover from a myocardial infarction. It is prudent to begin a program of gradually increasing exercise early in the course of the myocardial infarction, while the patient is hospitalized.

Obviously, the program must depend upon the condition of the patient, and it should be aimed toward complete rehabilitation. Walking, swimming or riding a bicycle are all perfectly satisfactory. Whatever the mode of exercise, it should be gradually increased and monitored by the patient's personal physician. After following such a program, the patient can perform more exercise at a lower pulse rate and blood pressure. If he has angina pectoris, keeping in good physical condition will enable him to be much more active before his heart reaches the point of myocardial oxygen consumption that results in chest pain. A patient must have the confidence not to unnecessarily limit his level of physical activity, because doing so will actually reduce the amount of exercise he can perform without having an anginal attack. Supervised conditioning at a gym or club is ideal, but if this is not practicable, the patient's physician can prescribe a safe program individualized to specific needs. Many of our patients have purchased a stationary bicycle which permits them to exercise in the comfort of their home.

We recommend assiduous attention to the correction of risk factors for our patients who have experienced a myocardial infarction. Our program involves giving up cigarette smoking; vigorous control of hypertension; correction of elevated serum cholesterol and triglyceride with diet and, if necessary, drugs; adjustment of diet to reach and maintain ideal body weight and as low a serum cholesterol as possible; regular exercise; and adjustment of life style to avoid excessive stress. These preventive measures are discussed in detail in Chapter 17.

In spite of medication and other precautions, however, angina pectoris cannot be satisfactorily controlled in many patients; in such cases surgical treatment is required.

Surgical Treatment

The surgical treatment for coronary artery disease began more than fifty years ago when Professor Thomas Jonnesco performed a sympathectomy (interrupting some of the nerve supply to the heart) to treat angina pectoris. This proved to be so successful that it caused great enthusiasm for surgical treatment of the sympathetic nervous system for coronary arterial disease. Although from time to time great enthusiasm developed for various procedures, surgeons subsequently lost interest, largely because of inconclusive and disappointing results.

In the early 1960s, there was a revival of interest in surgical treatment geared toward a direct approach to the problem. Two major factors were responsible for this breakthrough. The first was the development of coronary arteriography. Arteriography is the keystone for surgical treatment because it provides visualization of the arterial lumen, the precise location and the nature and extent of the obstruction. Indeed, this was the key that opened the door to surgical treatment for other forms of arterial disease in the early 1950s. But its safe application to the study of coronary arterial disease was delayed for about a decade.

The second major factor was concerned with the development of surgical procedures designed to restore normal circulation in an artery beyond an obstruction. Experience with the procedures developed for treating occlusive disease of the aorta and major arteries (see Chapter 6) encouraged surgeons to consider applying the techniques to similar lesions of the coronary arteries once coronary arteriography was developed as a safe diagnostic procedure.

In the first attempts to apply one of these direct surgical approaches, *endarterectomy* and patch graft angioplasty were used. While such procedures could be highly successful (indeed, we have some patients who are still living and doing well since their operation in the early 1960s), a high proportion—as many as one-half—were failures, and often the patient died following the operation. Considerable doubt arose about the future of a direct surgical approach.

This somewhat gloomy picture was changed by two important developments: the bypass technique and the heart-lung machine. In 1964 we performed the first coronary bypass using a segment of vein removed from the groin in a patient with severe angina pectoris. The operation was successful in restoring the patient to relatively normal activity. Since that time the procedure has been improved and perfected and the indications for its application have been more precisely defined through the investigation and experience of many surgeons across the country. It is now well established as the appropriate treatment for certain forms of coronary artery disease.

The selection of patients for surgical treatment depends on careful assessment of the cardiac function and precise arteriographic evaluation of the atherosclerotic occlusive process. Assessment of cardiac function is based on a detailed history from the patient, physical examination and special laboratory tests, including treadmill exercise testing. If these procedures indicate coronary artery disease and the patient has angina pectoris, coronary arteriography may be indicated. Other potential indications for coronary arteriography are atypical chest pain of undetermined origin, congestive heart failure of undetermined cause, angina after a myocardial infarction and valvular heart disease with chest pain.

Depending upon the results of these tests, surgical treatment may be recommended. Important factors in deciding whether to recommend surgery are the site and extent of the obstructing lesions (Figure 72), the function of the left ventricle and the general clinical condition of the patient. Particularly important is the nature of the obstructing process, which may produce varying degrees of narrowing or even total obstruction of the arterial lumen. Narrowing of more than 60 or 70 percent of the lumen is considered of significance in causing a decrease in blood flow. The extent or pattern of the blockage is particularly important. Fortunately, in many patients, the pattern tends to be localized, with a relatively normal artery distal to the lesion. Regardless of how severe or extensive the occluding lesion is, if there is a sufficiently normal distal arterial segment, it is possible to perform surgical treatment if left ventricular function is not too severely impaired.

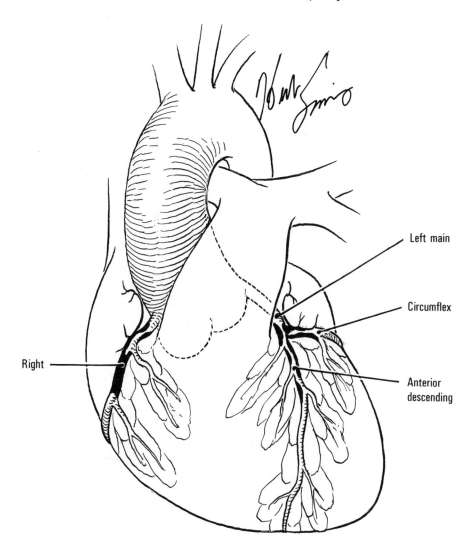

Figure 72. Patterns of coronary arterial disease

Therefore, surgical treatment is indicated for patients who have angina not adequately controlled by proper medical management; who have the pattern of occlusive disease characterized by a relatively normal artery beyond the occlusive process; and in whom left ventricular function is not too severely impaired. It may also be indicated in certain patients who are threatened with myocardial infarction termed preinfarctional, or crescendo, angina, and in some individuals who have a history of previous myocardial infarction and severe stenosis of the left main coronary artery or left anterior descending coronary artery. It is also indicated in patients with significant obstructive lesions of the coronary arteries who require surgical correction of valvular heart disease or an aneurysm of the left ventricle. It is occasionally indicated in patients with intractable cardiac arrhythmia. There may be other indications which involve special circumstances that require the professional judgment of the cardiologist and cardiac surgeon.

It is important to recognize that not all patients with coronary artery disease need or should have surgical treatment. Indeed, there are certain forms of the disease in which surgery is of no value or which are not amenable to surgical treatment. For example, patterns that are characterized by diffuse involvement, sometimes with calcification or with extensive narrowing of the distal arterial segments, do not lend themselves to surgical treatment. In instances when the muscle of the left ventricle is severely damaged or extensively scarred from previous myocardial infarction so that poor left ventricular function results, an operation usually is not indicated. In such patients the risk is very high and it is extremely doubtful that the patient will be much improved. Age, in itself, however, is not a contraindication to surgery. Our own experience and that of others has shown that properly selected patients in their seventies and eighties, who otherwise are in reasonably good general condition, may be successfully operated upon without a very high risk.

As mentioned before, the two basic surgical procedures used for the treatment of coronary occlusive disease are endarterectomy and bypass. Endarterectomy consists of removing the atheromatous process by separating it from the remainder of the arterial wall. It usually is applied only for extremely well-localized lesions. The operation is performed by making a longitudinal incision in the artery from well above to well below the occlusive lesion. A cleavage plane is then found between the atheromatous lesion and the remainder of the arterial wall and the lesion is separated carefully from the wall in a similar way as one would peel the covering of an orange from the inner fruit. The lesion is completely removed and the incision is closed by a fine suture or with a small patch (see Figures 40 and 41). Sometimes, if the proximal part of the artery is extensively blocked, it may be possible to perform endarterectomy using carbon dioxide gas to separate the atheroma from the arterial wall in the distal right coronary artery and then attach a bypass graft to the open distal segment (Figure 73). In the great majority of cases, however, the coronary artery disease does not lend itself to the procedure of endarterectomy.

The bypass operation has proved to be the procedure of choice in the great majority of patients for whom surgery is indicated. This operation is performed under general anesthesia using the heart-lung machine to support the patient during actual performance of the bypass. A segment of the saphenous vein, a fairly large superficial vein in the leg, is removed. Removal

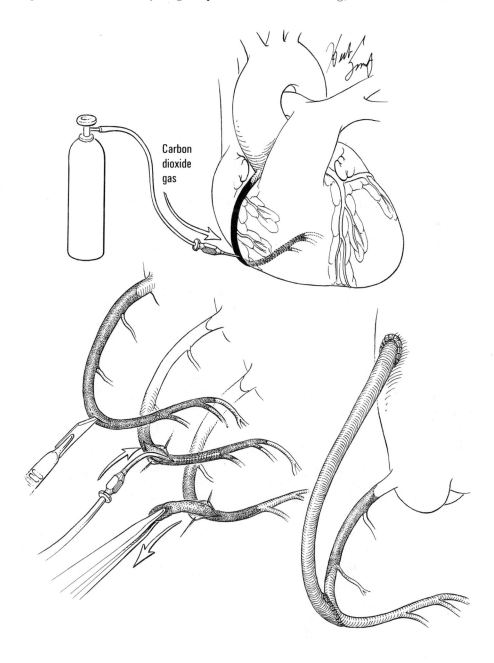

Carbon
dioxide
gas

Figure 73. Technique of carbon dioxide gas endarterectomy to open the distal right coronary artery before attachment of a bypass graft

of the vein causes no circulatory disturbances in the leg since there are sufficient other veins to replace its function. The vein graft is prepared by ligating, or closing off, its small branches. Because of its valves (see Figure 34), it will be attached so that blood will flow through it in the same direction as when it functioned in the leg. The heart is exposed by a median sternotomy, a longitudinal incision that is made through the breastbone using an electrical saw. Since the coronary arteries are on the surface of the heart, it is relatively easy to identify and isolate the proper segment for attachment of the graft as determined by the arteriogram. The patient is connected to the heart-lung machine and, in most instances, the heart function is stopped by occluding the ascending aorta and stopping blood flow to the heart through the coronary arteries. This is termed anoxic arrest and it provides a quiet heart which facilitates the delicate suture connection of a vein graft to a coronary artery. A longitudinal incision, about one-quarter inch in length, is made in a reasonably normal segment of the coronary artery beyond the obstructive lesion (Figure 74). The distal end of the graft is beveled and trimmed to fit the opening in the artery and then attached to the edges of the incision by a fine plastic suture. When the attachment is completed, the aortic clamp is removed to allow blood flow through the coronary arteries to resume. In a few seconds the heart starts to beat again. Sometimes the heart goes into ventricular fibrillation and requires an electrical shock to convert it to a normal rhythm. The heart is easily able to tolerate reduced blood flow for the fifteen minutes required to perform the anastomosis.

A special partial occlusion clamp is then applied to the anterior wall of the ascending aorta to isolate a part of its circumference while still allowing blood to flow through to beyond the pinched-off area. A longitudinal incision is then made in the isolated segment. The unattached end of the vein graft is tailored to fit this opening and then attached by a fine suture in a manner similar to the anastomosis of the distal end. Once this is completed, the partial occluding clamp on the ascending aorta is removed, allowing blood to flow through the vein into the distal coronary artery. Additional bypasses may be performed to other coronary arteries depending upon the nature and extent of occlusive lesions (Figure 75). Most patients require two, three or, occasionally, more bypasses. After completion of the bypass the patient is disconnected from the heart-lung machine and the incision is closed.

Results of the operation in terms of relief of chest pain are excellent. During the past decade we have performed more than ten thousand coronary bypass operations with highly gratifying results. The risk of operation is now only about 2 percent and more than 90 percent of the patients are significantly improved. Indeed, most of them are completely relieved of chest pain and resume normal activities. Some actually resume work that involves considerable physical activity. Long-term results are also excellent with recurrence of symptoms in only about 3 or 4 percent per year. The question

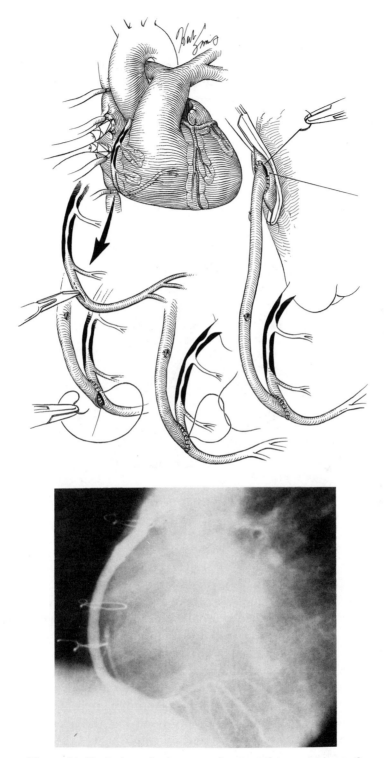

Figure 74. Technique for bypass using a saphenous vein graft from the aorta to the distal right coronary artery. Coronary arteriogram shows graft functioning five years after operation.

of whether or not the operation prolongs life is still undetermined, although there is some evidence to suggest that it does. While reduction of mortality is an important consideration, the primary reason for the operation is to relieve the patient of disabling symptoms and restore him to functional activity.

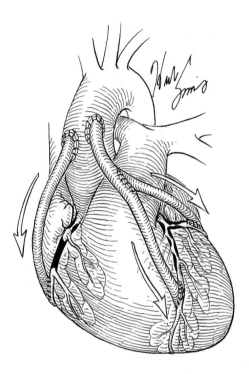

Figure 75. Vein grafts used to bypass occlusive disease in all three coronary arteries

Most patients with acute myocardial infarction can be adequately and successfully treated medically. Surgical treatment, however, may be recommended for some patients with severe infarction complicated by shock that resists medical treatment and is associated with severe arrhythmia. Under these circumstances the patient is usually placed on some type of mechanical heart support device, in most instances the intra-aortic balloon (see Figure 115) or the heart-lung machine, and an emergency coronary arteriogram is performed. If the pattern of the occlusive disease is amenable to surgical treatment, the patient is immediately taken to the operating room and the appropriate bypass operation is performed. Approximately 30 percent of such cases are successful. This may seem very poor, but the nearly 100 percent mortality rate in these patients without operation makes the relatively high risk of the operation acceptable.

Surgical treatment may also be suggested for patients who develop a left ventricular aneurysm after a myocardial infarction. This complication is produced by scar formation which replaces the damaged muscle of the left ventricle during the healing process. The scarred area is unable to resist the pounding pressure of repeated ventricular contraction. The weakened ventricular wall balloons out, sometimes growing larger than the left

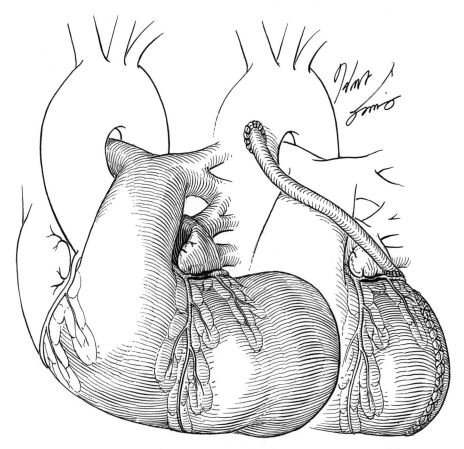

Figure 76. Left ventricular aneurysm following myocardial infarction (left) is treated by excision of the aneurysm. In some patients a vein graft may be placed from the aorta to the appropriate distal coronary artery (right).

ventricle itself. The aneurysm may ultimately rupture, but more frequently, the paradoxical motion of the aneurysm in opposition to the contracting ventricle interferes with left ventricular function and leads to heart failure. Under these circumstances surgery is recommended. With the patient supported by the heart-lung machine, the scarred area is excised and the opening in the left ventricle is repaired by suturing the edges together (Figure 76). In patients with occlusion of the coronary arteries, vein bypass also may be performed. Results of this operation are excellent with a better than 90 percent recovery rate.

Mitral insufficiency or incompetence of the mitral valve occurs as a complication of myocardial infarction when the heart is damaged at the site of attachment of the *chordae tendinae* from the *papillary muscles* (Figure 77). These are the stringlike attachments to the edges of the valve cusps which resemble the ropes attached to the edges of a parachute. Rupture of these attachments following infarction allows the cusp of the mitral valve to flop back and forth uselessly, and often results in heart failure. Surgical treatment usually consists of replacing the damaged valve with an artificial one and sometimes placing a vein bypass to the coronary arteries. Results of the operation are quite good, with a relatively low risk.

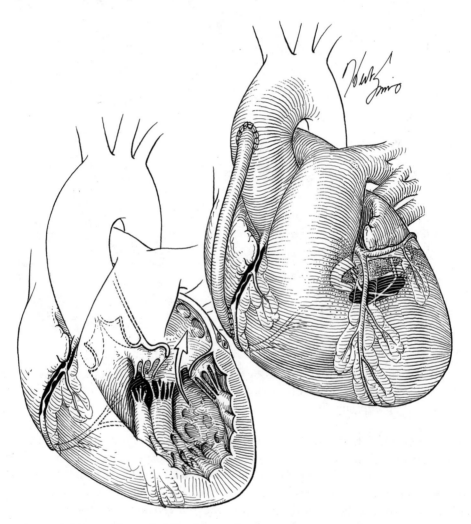

Figure 77. Incompetence of the mitral valve occurring as a complication of myocardial infarction (left) is treated by valve replacement. In some patients a bypass graft may be placed to the appropriate distal coronary artery (right).

Ventricular septal defect may also be a complication of myocardial infarction (Figure 78). This occurs from infarction damage to the ventricular septum and death of the tissues so that they are no longer able to tolerate the pressure in the left ventricle. If the resulting opening is large enough, the patient develops acute, severe heart failure that usually is fatal. Surgical correction of the defect, usually with a Dacron patch, is performed in much the same manner as for congenital ventricular septal defects and results of the operation are reasonably good.

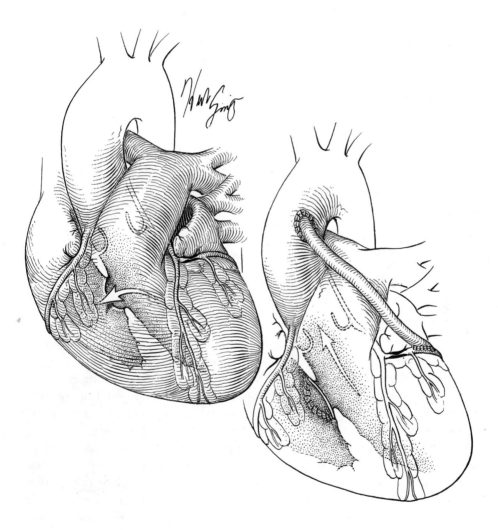

Figure 78. Ventricular septal defect occurring as a complication of myocardial infarction (left) is treated by closing of the defect with a Dacron graft. In some patients a bypass graft may be placed to the appropriate distal coronary artery (right).

10

STROKE

THE first successful carotid endarterectomy on a stroke patient was performed by Dr. Michael DeBakey at the Cardiovascular Center of The Methodist Hospital on August 7, 1953. This patient survived nineteen years with no recurrence of any stroke symptoms and ultimately died of coronary artery disease. At the time of this operation, the concept underlying cerebrovascular insufficiency, or lack of circulation to the brain caused by occlusive disease in the major arteries supplying blood to the brain, had not yet been established. However, certain studies suggested that such lesions might cause some strokes. The successful surgical treatment of this patient helped to confirm that localized occlusive disease in the carotid artery of the neck was one of the major causes of the symptoms of stroke, and that removal of the obstructing lesion with restoration of normal circulation in the artery was an effective method of treatment. This gratifying experience provided much encouragement for a more intensive investigation of the problem.

It is interesting that the risk of stroke in the black male is about five times as great as in the white male, while the risk of dying from a myocardial

144

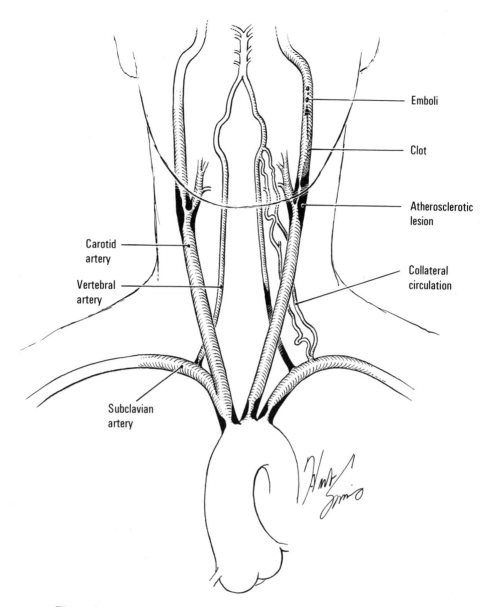

Figure 79. Patterns of occlusive disease in the major arteries supplying blood to the brain. A clot may form at one of these lesions, and pieces may break off to form emboli, which can pass through the bloodstream to block important vessels in the brain, causing a stroke. During slow onset of an occlusive lesion, collateral circulation may develop to provide for the flow of blood around the occluded artery.

infarction is five times greater in white males. The increased mortality from cerebrovascular disease in blacks is likely explained, in part, by a higher incidence in blacks of hypertension, the single most important risk factor for stroke and, particularly, for cerebral hemorrhage.

Findings from the International Atherosclerosis Project show that blacks have more atherosclerotic involvement of the intracranial arteries than whites, while whites have more extensive atheromatous disease of the aorta and coronary arteries. A similar relationship exists between Japanese and American Caucasians, again likely on the basis of a higher incidence of hypertension in Japan.

There are a number of different causes of stroke, but one of the most important and common is obstruction of blood flow to the brain which results from arteriosclerosis or atherosclerosis (Figure 79). Eventually the lumen of the artery becomes so narrowed that it does not let enough blood through to nourish the area of the brain it serves. Moreover, the blood flow now becomes sluggish enough to lead to the formation of a blood clot that then completely obstructs the artery. This type of stroke is called a cerebral thrombosis.

Another common cause of stroke is cerebral hemorrhage, which is usually associated with hypertension. It is caused by a tear in the diseased artery which results in bleeding into the brain.

A third cause of stroke results from an embolus, which consists of a small clot or even part of the atheromatous material in the arterial wall that breaks off and is then swept up by the bloodstream to lodge in a small artery blocking circulation. There are still other causes, such as congenital vascular malformations, aneurysms, and even traumas. Our major concern here is with those forms of stroke caused by arteriosclerotic or atherosclerotic occlusive disease of the major arteries to the brain which are amenable to surgical treatment.

As you may recall there are four major arteries supplying blood to the brain. Three arteries arise from the aortic arch, which receives most of the blood pumped out by the heart. The first of the three large arteries which spring from the aortic arch is the innominate, which divides at the base of the neck into the right subclavian and right common carotid arteries. The second major artery originating from the aortic arch is the left common carotid artery and the third is the left subclavian artery. Each of the two common carotid arteries divides just below the angle of the jaw into two major branches, the external carotid artery supplying blood to the neck and face, and the internal carotid artery that continues upward to enter the skull through a small opening and supplies blood to the eyes and the brain. Two other major vessels that supply blood to the brain are called the vertebral arteries, which arise from the right and left subclavian arteries. After entering the skull, the two vertebral arteries usually join to form the basilar artery at the base of the brain. In addition to these four main arteries, there are several smaller arterial connections between them both inside and outside of the skull. These are termed collateral arteries because they provide an alternate route for the circulation. They may assume great importance in a patient who develops a stroke from obstruction of one of the four major arteries, since they are sometimes able to shunt enough blood around the blockage to sustain the area of the brain supplied by the obstructed artery. This is one of the reasons some patients completely recover from a stroke without any treatment. Such complete recovery, however, occurs in only a small number of patients, since, in most cases, collateral circulation is not sufficient to provide a normal blood flow. It may, however, help to maintain viability of the brain until normal circulation is restored and thus permit enough time for surgical treatment.

A particularly important consideration in determining treatment is the nature and location of the obstructing lesions in the arteries supplying blood to the brain. In the great majority of cases, these occlusive lesions are well localized to certain segments of the arteries, often not more than one-half to a little more than one inch in length, and the remainder of the artery above and below the lesion is normal. The most common location of these obstructive lesions is in the common carotid arteries where they divide into the external and internal carotid arteries just below the angle of the jaw. The next most common site is in the vertebral arteries just as they arise from the subclavian arteries. The third most common location is in the innominate, left common carotid and left subclavian arteries near their origin from the aortic arch. Arteriosclerosis or atherosclerosis is most often the cause of these patterns. However, a nonarteriosclerotic type of obstructive lesion may occur here which is called arteritis. It is a peculiar inflammatory condition and tends to occur mostly in young female patients. Fortunately, in both types of lesion, the obstruction tends to be well localized, with relatively normal arteries distal to the obstruction. About one-half of the patients have only one of the four major arteries affected; of the remaining patients, two or more of these arteries are affected.

Arteriosclerotic or atherosclerotic occlusive disease of the carotid and vertebral arteries occurs most commonly in males between the ages of fifty and seventy years. Symptoms vary considerably, depending upon the extent of obstruction and the arteries involved. In general, a decrease in blood flow from obstruction of the internal carotid artery produces symptoms resulting from functional impairment of the front part of the brain—the area concerned with memory, control of muscular movements and the appreciation of sensations such as touch, temperature and pain. A variety of symptoms may then occur including weakness, paralysis, numbness and tingling on the side of the body opposite the occluded vessel, since each side of the brain controls the opposite side of the body. However, in most people speech is controlled by the left side of the brain and is, therefore, usually only affected by obstruction of the left internal carotid artery.

Atherosclerotic lesions of the carotid artery also may produce strokelike symptoms by a process other than actual obstruction of blood flow. In such cases the lesion may be ulcerated on its inner surface with deposits of a thrombus or clot. Small particles of this clotted material, or even of the cholesterol and fatty deposition in the atheromatous lesion, may break off and then be swept up in the bloodstream to block circulation to a segment of the brain. This is called embolization, and symptoms of this type of occlusion usually come on suddenly. Again, depending upon the adequacy of collateral circulation, symptoms may be transient, with complete recovery.

Symptoms produced by vertebral artery obstruction may be extremely variable, depending upon the section of the brain affected by the inadequate circulation. The vertebral arteries supply blood to the upper part of the spinal cord, the base and back part of the brain, and the cerebellum. Since, for example, the back part of the brain controls vision, the patient may have difficulty in seeing. Such visual disturbances usually occur in both eyes in contrast to patients with obstruction of the internal carotid artery who will have difficulty with only one eye. Inadequate circulation to the cerebellum produces symptoms of vertigo, or dizziness, and inability to perform fine, delicately coordinated movements. Impaired blood flow to the base of the brain produces disturbances in sensation and weakness or paralysis on both sides of the body, rather than on one side as occurs in obstruction of the internal carotid artery.

The pattern, variety and severity of symptoms depend upon a number of factors, particularly the site and severity of obstruction, the number of arteries affected and the amount of blood supplied by collateral circulation. If, for example, the artery is not completely blocked, there may be enough circulation through it and through collateral circulation to maintain normal function most of the time. Symptoms may, however, be precipitated by several contributing factors, such as a reduction in blood pressure, which further reduces the flow of blood through the partially blocked artery. Reduced blood pressure may occur from drugs, a shift in position from lying to sitting to standing, or changes in heart function. The patient may then have brief attacks or small strokes during which he experiences slight weakness or even paralysis, difficulty in speech or partial blindness. He may recover completely in a few seconds, minutes or hours. In spite of this recovery, such seizures often precede further attacks which may ultimately result in permanent brain damage or even death.

Obstruction of the main arteries arising from the aortic arch, i.e. the innominate, common carotid and subclavian arteries, produces a wide variety of symptoms, since the entire brain receives its blood supply from these major arteries. Because two of these vessels—the left subclavian and the innominate, which gives rise to the right subclavian artery—supply blood to the arms as well as the brain, obstructive lesions in these arteries may produce inadequate circulation to the arms, resulting in cramps in the arms or hands during exercise, and coldness and pain in the hands and fingers. In rare cases, even gangrene of the fingers may occur. When such symptoms are accompanied by the absence of a pulse at the wrist, or diminished blood pressure in one or both arms, the obstructions are in the subclavian arteries.

The diagnosis of obstructive or ulcerative lesions can usually be suspected from the symptoms of the patient and further confirmed by a careful physical and neurological examination. Although not always present, a particularly significant sign of occlusive lesions in the carotid artery is the presence of a bruit, or murmur, heard through a stethoscope placed on the neck just below the angle of the jaw. This is a swishing noise, synchronized with the heartbeat, and is produced by the blood as it rushes through the narrowed part of the artery. Sometimes the patient himself may hear the sound in his own ear.

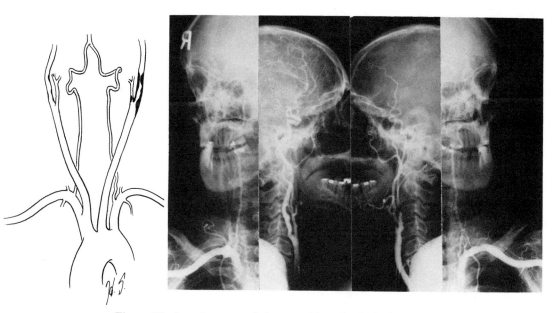

Figure 80. Arteriograms of the carotid and subclavian arteries provide precise information about occlusive lesion in the arteries supplying blood to the brain.

After the patient has been thoroughly evaluated by a clinical and neurological examination that indicates the probable diagnosis of occlusive disease, a precise diagnosis can then be made by arteriography (Figure 80). The procedure can be performed under local or light general anesthesia. Carotid and subclavian arteriography accurately shows the location of the obstruction and also provides information necessary for determining the need and the type of surgical treatment. In our experience with thousands of cases at the Cardiovascular Center of The Methodist Hospital, the risk is extremely small (about one per thousand) and there are few complications.

Treatment may be medical or surgical, depending upon a number of factors. Usually surgical treatment is recommended for well-localized obstructive or ulcerative lesions of the carotid artery, obstructive lesions involving the origin of the vertebral arteries, and in occlusive lesions of the

major arteries arising from the aortic arch. Surgery may also be suggested for
some patients with severe obstructive lesions of the internal carotid artery in
the neck who are relatively asymptomatic. These are usually patients who are
found to have such a lesion on routine examination, or who may require an
operation for another related condition. In our early experience we encountered some patients who developed a stroke following other operations, and
were subsequently found to have an obstructive lesion of the internal carotid
artery which could have been surgically corrected before the operation,
possibly precluding the development of the stroke. On the basis of this
experience it is now our practice to perform arteriograms on patients who
have significant murmurs, or bruits over the carotid artery, and if the
arteriogram demonstrates a severe occlusive lesion, surgical treatment is
recommended.

Surgical treatment is not routine for all patients with occlusive disease of
the arteries supplying blood to the brain. Operations are not recommended
for patients with occlusive lesions of the arteries within the skull nor for

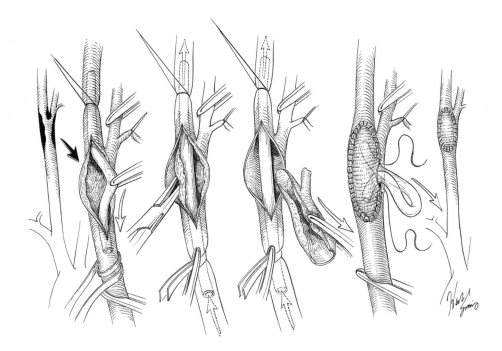

Figure 81. Endarterectomy and patch-graft angioplasty may
be used to treat occlusive disease in the bifurcation of the
carotid artery. A temporary shunt is placed to provide blood
to the brain during the procedure. The lesion is peeled away
from the arterial wall and a Dacron patch is sewn in the
opening. The shunt is withdrawn before the suture is tied.

patients with complete occlusion of the major arteries in the neck who have a permanent condition such as paralysis or develop a speech defect after a period of weeks or months. Under these circumstances the brain damage is not reversible even if circulation can be restored, although surgery may be performed in such cases as an emergency procedure within six to twelve hours after the stroke occurs. This decision to operate requires careful assessment by the neurologist and the surgeon. Certain associated diseases, such as severe emphysema or heart failure, and some debilitating conditions may also discourage surgical treatment because of the high risk of operation.

Restoration of circulation is accomplished by one of two types of operation, namely *thromboendarterectomy* and the bypass graft principle. In occlusive and ulcerative lesions involving the common carotid artery and the origin of the internal carotid artery, the procedure of endarterectomy is usually performed (Figure 81). These lesions are well localized within a short segment of the artery and it is possible to separate the lesion cleanly from the remainder of the arterial wall. The artery is exposed through a small incision in the neck and temporary occluding clamps are applied above and below the lesion. An incision is made through the wall of the artery just below the blockage and continued up through the obstructed segment for a short distance into the healthy artery. A temporary shunt consisting of a small plastic tube is then inserted into the opening above and below the obstruction to allow blood to flow to the brain while the operation is being performed. The diseased lesion, termed an atheroma, is then removed by separating it cleanly from its attachment to the arterial wall. The incision in the artery is then closed by sewing the edges together with a fine suture or in some cases, because this may produce some reduction in the bore of the artery, a small patch of Dacron fabric is sutured to the edges as a patch graft. Just before completing the closure, the internal plastic tube shunt is removed and the final closure is completed. In time, a new intimal lining covers the entire area, including the inner surface of the graft.

In obstructing lesions of the major arteries arising from the aortic arch, the bypass principle is preferred. In virtually all such cases the obstructive lesions are well localized, with relatively normal arteries beyond the obstruction in the neck. This, of course, is the reason the bypass graft can be applied so successfully in these cases. The operation is performed by exposing the ascending aorta through a small incision at the front of the chest on the right side, usually between the second and third ribs. Using a special partial occluding clamp, a small portion of the ascending aorta is pinched off and an incision is made through the wall of the vessel in this pinched-off segment. A tubular Dacron graft is attached to this opening by sewing the edges of the graft to the edges of the opening in the aorta. The graft is then passed up into the base of the neck through a tunnel made in the tissue at the front of the neck where it joins the chest. The appropriate artery beyond the obstruction is exposed by an incision in the neck. The other end of the Dacron tube is attached to an opening made in the artery where it is relatively healthy, by a similar suture procedure. In this way blood is shunted from the ascending aorta to the artery beyond its obstruction, thus restoring normal circulation to the brain (Figure 82). In some cases in which more than one of these major

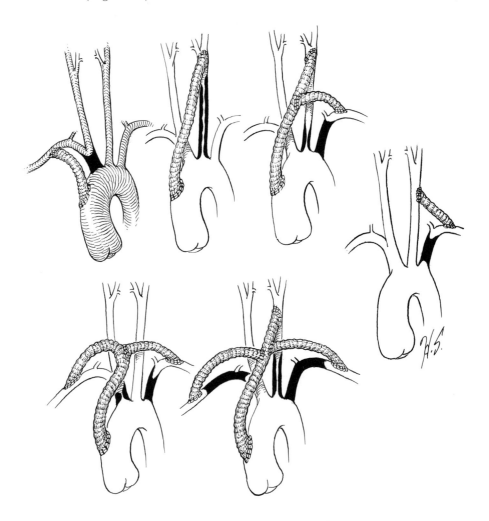

Figure 82. Examples of some of the varieties of bypass grafts
that can be used as a treatment of occlusive lesion in the
proximal arteries arising from the aortic arch

arteries is obstructed, additional grafts may be attacked to the main graft from the ascending aorta. In instances where the occlusive lesion is limited to the subclavian artery, an even simpler operation may be done by employing a bypass graft from the healthy common carotid artery to the subclavian artery beyond the obstruction through an incision exposing both arteries in the neck.

Results of these operations have been extremely gratifying. The risk of operation is only about 1 or 2 percent, and complications are also minimal—about 2 percent. Long-term results have also been good. Postoperative follow-up studies extending from ten to twenty years have demonstrated that the great majority of patients are completely relieved of symptoms and have few recurrences.

11

OCCLUSIVE
DISEASE

Occlusive Disease of the Lower Extremities

Arteriosclerosis or atherosclerosis is the underlying lesion in the great majority of patients with occlusive disease of the lower extremities. The disease tends to assume distinctive patterns of location and extent. It may be completely confined to the terminal abdominal aorta and its major branches, the common iliac arteries, with relatively normal arteries below (Figure 83). This pattern of the disease is often termed the Leriche syndrome, after the late French surgeon René Leriche who originally described it. As the atheromatous process progresses, it narrows the lumen of the aorta or iliac arteries, decreasing blood flow and ultimately causing complete obstruction. A second pattern of the disease involves the main arteries in the thighs, the superficial femoral arteries. Here again, the disease is localized, usually in the mid-portion of the thigh, with relatively normal arteries above and below. The disease begins with a gradual narrowing of the lumen of the artery and progresses to complete obstruction, sometimes because of clotting. In some

154

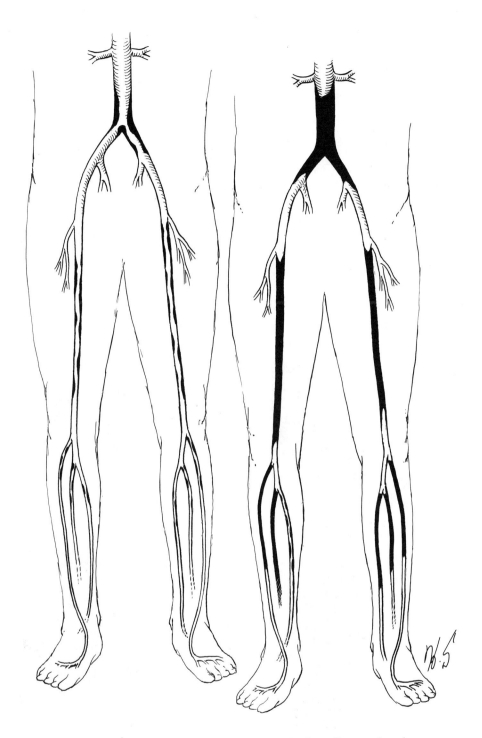

Figure 83. Typical patterns of occlusive disease in the abdominal aorta and vessels to the legs. Diffuse lesions which partially block the vessels (left) may progress to total occlusion (right).

patients there is a combination of these two patterns with localized involvement in the abdominal aorta, iliac arteries and superficial femoral arteries in the thighs. Still another pattern of the disease involves the arteries below the knee. This is the most serious pattern because it does not lend itself to effective treatment.

Occlusive disease of the lower extremities occurs most often in men (in a ratio of about ten to one) usually between the ages of forty and seventy. It may, however, occur in patients in their twenties or in some over eighty years of age. In women it occurs more frequently after the age of sixty.

Symptoms depend upon the site and extent of the disease and its speed of development. If the disease develops gradually, allowing time for collateral circulation to occur, symptoms are minimal at first and progress slowly. If the disease strikes without time for development of collateral circulation, impairment of distal circulation may occur quite suddenly. Most patients, however, develop symptoms gradually. In patients with the aorto-iliac pattern of the disease, the most common complaint is pain in the buttocks, thighs and lower extremities during exercise. It is characterized by relief

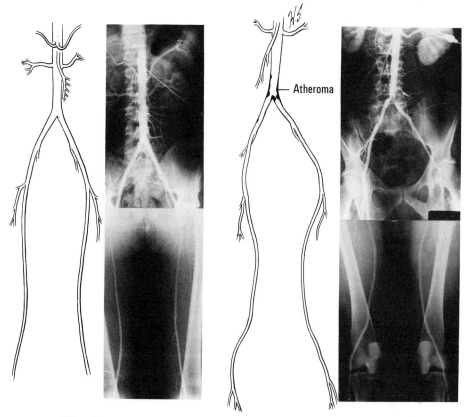

Figure 84. Aortography provides information about the exact site and extent of occlusive disease in the aorta and its major branches.

when resting and renewed pain when walking or exercising. This is termed *intermittent claudication*. With the gradual progression of the disease, the patient finds that he can walk only a few blocks or less before the pain becomes so severe that he must stop and rest before walking again. Often the aorto-iliac pattern of the disease causes male patients to become impotent. Patients whose superficial femoral arteries in the thighs are affected complain of tighteninglike pain in the calves of the legs during walking or exercise. As both patterns of the disease worsen, claudication becomes more severe, the ability to walk becomes more limited and there eventually is pain even at rest. There is a simultaneous atrophy of the muscles in the legs, wasting of the subcutaneous tissues, coldness of the feet, loss of hair and excessive growth of the toenails. Ultimately, gangrenous changes may occur in the skin of the feet and toes, often precipitated by a slight injury.

The diagnosis usually is made from the typical symptoms described above, along with the diminution or absence of pulses in the lower extremities. However, arteriography is required to provide more precise information, particularly to determine the pattern of the disease so the most appropriate therapy can be selected. Arteriography is performed by the injection of a radiopaque substance into the aorta or artery above the occlusive process, followed by an x-ray. This procedure permits visualization of the normal lumen of the aorta and its major branches and the exact site and extent of the occlusive lesion (Figure 84). The risk involved with this

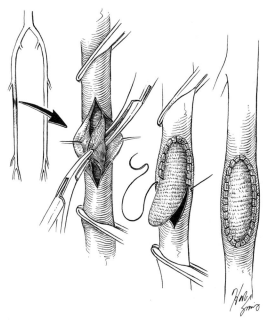

Figure 85. Technique of endarterectomy and patch-graft angioplasty to treat a localized lesion of the superficial femoral artery

procedure is extremely low, as evidenced by our experience in which significant complications have occurred in only one patient out or three or four thousand.

Treatment is directed toward restoration of normal circulation by one of several surgical procedures, depending upon the pattern of the disease. One procedure used is *thromboendarterectomy,* which consists of removing the atheromatous lesion by dissecting or separating it from the arterial wall (Figure 85). The incision in the artery is often repaired by using a patch in order to avoid constriction of the lumen after closing the incision. This technique is used in extremely well-localized lesions, perhaps no more than an inch or two in length.

A second method is the application of a bypass graft. In the great

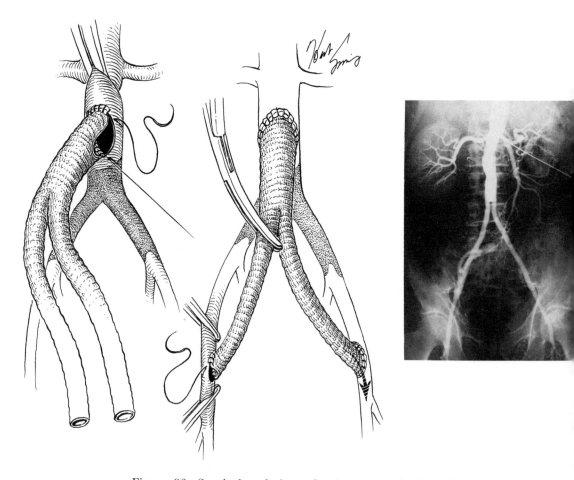

Figure 86. Surgical technique for bypass graft from the abdominal aorta to the femoral arteries. Aortogram shows graft functioning with restoration of normal circulation twenty years after operation.

majority of cases in our experience with disease of the terminal abdominal aorta and common iliac arteries, the bypass graft procedure has been found to be the most satisfactory. The trunk of a Y-shaped Dacron graft is attached to an opening made in the aorta above the obstructive lesion, usually just below the origin of the renal arteries (Figure 86). The two limbs of the graft are attached by end to side anastomosis to the main arteries below the obstruction. By this means, circulation is shunted through the graft around the obstructed segment and into the arteries of the lower extremities.

Results of the operation are excellent, with successful restoration of circulation in about 98 percent of the patients. Long-term results are good; many patients maintain relatively normal and even vigorous physical activity for ten to twenty years. The risk of operation is minimal, with an operative mortality of only 1 or 2 percent.

For the second pattern of disease, in which the superficial femoral artery in the thigh is involved, the bypass procedure also has been found to be the most satisfactory (Figure 87). In this procedure a small incision is made in the groin to expose the common femoral artery and a longitudinal incision is made in the artery between temporary occluding clamps. One end of a Dacron graft is attached to this opening by end to side anastomosis. The vessel below the obstruction, the *popliteal artery,* then is exposed by an incision on the inner side of the leg just above the knee. The other end of the graft is brought down to this incision through a tunnel under the skin and attached to an opening made in the popliteal artery. Circulation is thus shunted through the graft into the main artery of the lower leg. In some cases, particularly when the obstructive lesion extends for a short distance below the knee, it may be preferable to use a vein removed from the leg as the substitute artery instead of a Dacron graft.

Results of the operation are excellent, with restoration of circulation and normal activities in over 90 percent of the patients. The risk of operation is quite small, with an operative mortality rate of less than one percent.

In some patients with a combination of aorto-iliac and superficial femoral occlusive disease, it may be desirable to use both types of grafts. In other cases, the procedure of lumbar sympathectomy may be employed in conjunction with the use of the bypass graft. The procedure of sympathectomy consists of excising a small segment of the lumbar sympathetic nerve ganglia in order to interrupt the nerve impulses which cause constriction of the muscle in the wall of the arteries of the lower extremities. Its purpose is to permit a widening of the lumen of the arteries, particularly the smaller arteries, and thus to allow more blood to flow through these small arteries and a greater degree of collateral circulation to develop in the lower leg. Selection of the method of treatment is best made on an individual basis based on the type, nature and extent of the obstructive disease. Men should be aware of the possibility of being unable to ejaculate following the bilateral lumbar sympathectomy.

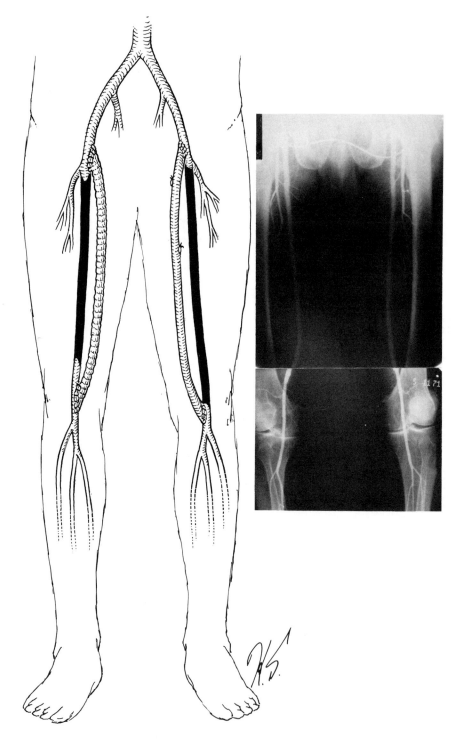

Figure 87. Occlusive disease of the superficial femoral arteries treated by a Dacron bypass graft in the right leg and vein graft in the left leg. Arteriogram shows a Dacron graft functioning ten years after operation.

With the third pattern of occlusive disease, the type in which the obstructive process involves the major arteries below the knee with relatively little or no occlusion in the arteries above this level, it is usually not possible to perform effective treatment by endarterectomy or the use of a bypass graft. Occasionally, the procedure of lumbar sympathectomy may provide some improvement.

Occlusive Disease of the Arteries to the Abdominal Organs

The arterial blood supply to the abdominal organs, such as the liver, spleen, stomach, intestines and kidneys, comes from arteries that arise from the abdominal aorta. Thus, the kidneys receive their blood supply from two arteries, termed the right and left renal arteries. The remaining abdominal organs receive their blood supply from the celiac, superior mesenteric and inferior mesenteric arteries. Aside from congenital abnormalities, such as coarctation (discussed in Chapter 7), certain acquired diseases may occur in these arteries causing disturbances in circulation and function.

There are two major causes of occlusive disease in the renal arteries. The first and by far the most common is atherosclerosis, which usually is well localized in the proximal portion of the artery, with a relatively normal distal segment (Figure 88). The second, which is much rarer, is termed *fibromuscular*

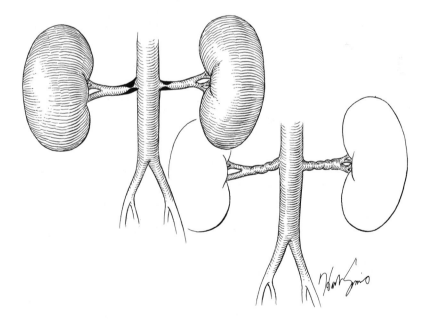

Figure 88. Patterns of occlusive disease of renal arteries with atherosclerotic occlusive disease (left) and fibromuscular hyperplasia (right)

hyperplasia, and is characterized by multiple areas of thickening of the middle layer of the arterial wall and, consequently, a narrowing of the lumen. This condition occurs most frequently in young women in their twenties and thirties. A most important consideration in both of these occlusive lesions is the fact that they are often associated with hypertension. This is believed to be caused by the diminution in blood flow and pulse pressure, triggering the production of the chemical renin in the kidney, as discussed in Chapter 14. Experience has shown that a casual relationship does exist in many patients with hypertension and renal artery occlusive lesions. It should be stated, however, that there are patients who develop these occlusive lesions but do not have hypertension.

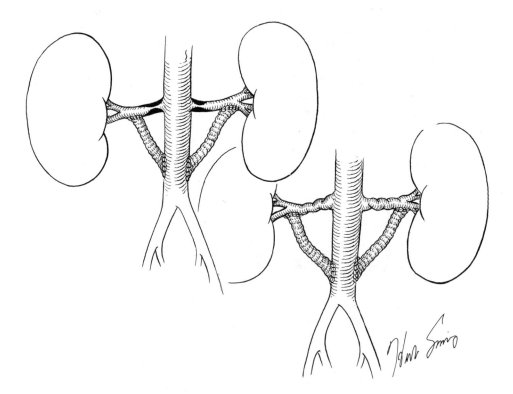

Figure 89. Bypass grafts used to bypass atherosclerotic occlusive lesions of the renal arteries (left) and occlusion by fibromuscular hyperplasia (right)

Atherosclerotic occlusive disease of the renal arteries occurs predominantly in men, and most frequently between the ages of fifty and seventy. Associated arteriosclerotic disease involving other major arteries of the body occurs in about one-third of these patients, and involvement of both renal arteries occurs in about one-third of the patients. A history of sudden onset of hypertension or of unresponsiveness to antihypertensive drugs suggests the possibility of occlusive disease in the renal arteries. The diagnosis usually can be made by special laboratory tests of kidney function and confirmed by arteriography, which shows the location and extent of the occlusive lesion. Evaluation of renal hypertension is discussed in Chapter 14.

The treatment is surgical and consists of either nephrectomy (removal of the diseased kidney) in cases in which the occlusion of the renal artery has extensively damaged the kidney, or restoration of normal circulation to the kidney, which may be achieved by either endarterectomy with patch graft angioplasty, or with a bypass graft. In the majority of cases, the bypass graft technique is preferred (Figure 89). A Dacron graft is attached to the abdominal aorta by end to side anastomosis and then to the renal artery just distal to the occlusive lesion.

Results are excellent, with an operative mortality of about 1 or 2 percent. In our experience with more than 1,600 cases, blood pressure was effectively reduced in 86 percent of the cases, and actually reached normal level in 57 percent of the cases. In some patients, the presence of longstanding hypertension had produced irreversible damage to the kidney so that surgical treatment did not cure or improve the elevation of blood pressure.

The clinical syndrome of abdominal angina (also termed chronic mesenteric vascular insufficiency, intestinal angina or splanchnic ischemia) usually is caused by atherosclerotic occlusive disease involving the celiac, superior mesenteric and inferior mesenteric arteries which supply blood to the gastrointestinal tract. In most patients, the atheromatous lesion is well localized in these arteries just beyond their origin from the aorta. In most patients suffering from symptoms of this type of disease, at least two of the arteries are involved, and sometimes all three.

The disease, in our clinical experience, is relatively rare, as evidenced by the fact that our own series of cases has been limited to about fifty. Occlusion of the celiac and mesenteric arteries occurs most often between the ages of fifty and seventy. The chief complaint is cramplike pain in the upper abdomen shortly after meals. This pain may last for several hours and often radiates to the back. Because the patient associates the pain with eating, he tends to eat less and, consequently, significant weight loss occurs. He may also complain of bloating, diarrhea, constipation, nausea and vomiting. Associated arteriosclerotic disease in other arteries of the body is not uncommon. The diagnosis is made by arteriography demonstrating the occlusive lesions.

Treatment is surgical and is directed toward restoring normal circulation in the affected arteries. In our experience, the bypass graft procedure has been found to be the most satisfactory (Figure 90). Because the occlusive lesion is usually well localized, with a relatively normal artery beyond the lesion, it is possible to attach a Dacron graft from the abdominal aorta to the distal artery. Blood is thereby shunted through the graft to the celiac and superior mesenteric arteries beyond the occlusive lesions. Results of this type of operation, which restores normal circulation to the gastrointestinal tract, have provided excellent relief of the patient's symptoms.

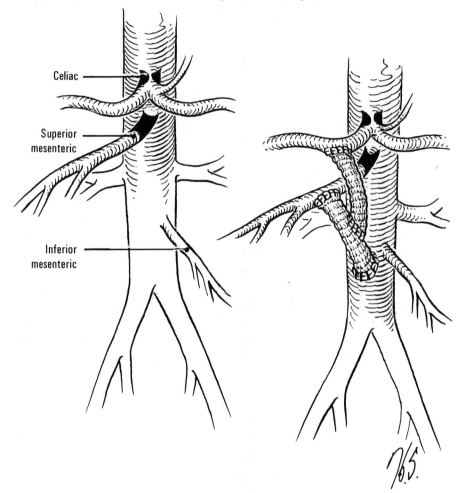

Celiac

Superior
mesenteric

Inferior
mesenteric

Figure 90. Use of Dacron bypass grafts to treat occlusive
lesions of celiac and superior mesenteric arteries

In advanced cases, where irreversible hypoxic damage to the bowel has occurred, the results are much less favorable and the mortality rate is quite high. Irreversible shock, gangrene of the bowel and peritonitis may occur in terminal cases resulting from ischemia of the bowel.

12

ANEURYSMS

T_{HE} term *aneurysm* is derived from the Greek word which means
to widen or dilate. It is a disease that has been known for centuries, and long
recognized as a threat to life. It develops from a weakness or destruction of
the media layer of the aorta or a major artery. Once this occurs, the
weakened part of the arterial wall gives way to the pounding pulse pressure
within the artery and enlarges (Figure 91). Ultimately, lethal complications
occur, either due to compression of surrounding structures or from rupture of
the aneurysm and *exsanguination.*

No effective treatment for aneurysm was available until relatively
recently. Beginning in the early 1950s, effective methods for surgical
treatment of aneurysms were developed and refined. It may now be stated
from a technical standpoint that virtually all aneurysms of the aorta and
major arteries can be effectively treated with a high rate of success.

Aneurysms are classified according to cause, location and morphology.
By far the most common cause is arteriosclerosis. It is not known why
arteriosclerosis in some patients affects the media layer of an artery leading to

165

aneurysm formation, and in others affects the intima leading to obstruction of the lumen. Indeed, in some patients both types of arterial disease are present in different parts of the arterial tree. Less frequently, aneurysms are caused by specific infections, particularly syphilis, which was one of the most

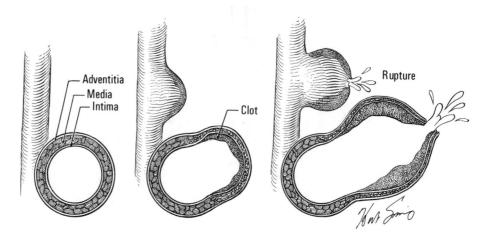

Figure 91. A normal artery (left) is weakened by arteriosclerosis or atherosclerosis and gradually balloons out, forming an aneurysm which may be partially lined with a blood clot (center). Eventually the aneurysm may rupture (right).

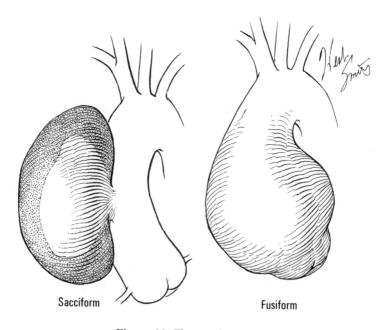

Figure 92. Types of aneurysms

common causes in earlier years before effective treatment for the disease was available; trauma; blunt injuries to the chest, often resulting from an automobile accident or from a fall; congential lesions; and a special form of disease of the media.

Morphologically, aneurysms may be classified into two types: 1) *fusiform,* characterized by involvement of the entire circumference of the aorta with a tendency to assume a spindle shape; and 2) *sacciform,* characterized by a pouchlike protrusion with a narrow neck from the arterial wall (Figure 92).

Aneurysms tend to assume distinctive localized patterns in terms of their extent and location, with relatively normal segments above and below. The most common pattern is an aneurysm of the abdominal aorta which arises just below the renal arteries and extends down to encompass the common iliac arteries (Figure 93). Next in frequency are aneurysms of the descending

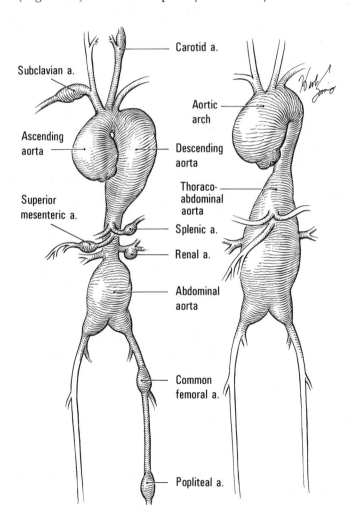

Figure 93. The anatomic locations of aneurysms

thoracic aorta, which arise just distal to the left subclavian artery and extend to the middle or lower third of the descending thoracic aorta, and sometimes to the diaphragm. Next are the aneurysms of the ascending aorta, the aortic arch and the thoracoabdominal aorta. Aneurysms of the other major arteries most frequently involve the common femoral artery in the groin, the popliteal artery behind the knee, the carotid artery in the neck and the subclavian arteries. Occasionally aneurysms occur in the renal arteries, the splenic artery and the superior mesenteric artery.

Aneurysm of the Abdominal Aorta

This is the most common type of aneurysm of the aorta and is caused by arteriosclerosis in the great majority of cases. It is also one of the most lethal, causing death from rupture in a high percentage of the patients. Studies of the natural history of the disease showed that about one-half of the patients died within one year after diagnosis and less than 10 percent survived for five years. The disease may occur anytime from the teens to the nineties, but the highest incidence occurs in people in their sixties and seventies. Men are affected in a ratio of nine to one over women. In about one-third of the patients there is associated hypertension and occlusive vascular disease in the arteries to the brain or the coronary arteries.

Symptoms may not occur at all, and the disease often is found during a routine physical examination. Sometimes the patient himself becomes aware of a prominent pulsation in the abdomen. Pain is a danger signal since it usually indicates progressive expansion with an imminent danger of leakage or rupture. The location and severity of pain depends upon the nature and extent of the aneurysm. It may be located in the back or radiate into the flanks, groin, testicles or legs. If leakage or rupture takes place, the pain may become more intense and the patient will develop a rapid heartbeat, sweating and shock. If a sudden rupture occurs, the patient may die within a few minutes.

The diagnosis can usually be made by a physical examination and x-rays of the abdomen. In questionable cases, aortography may be necessary.

Once the diagnosis is made, surgical treatment is recommended and consists of resection or removal of the aneurysm between occluding clamps and replacement with a Dacron graft. A Y-shaped graft is used if the aneurysm involves the common iliac arteries (Figure 94).

Results of the operation are quite good, with an operative risk of only about 2 or 3 percent and excellent long-term results. Some of our patients are leading a normal life twenty years after the operation. Contraindications to elective operation may include severe debilitating disease such as cancer, emphysema and heart failure. Age itself is not a negative factor, since we have successfully operated on patients in their eighties and nineties.

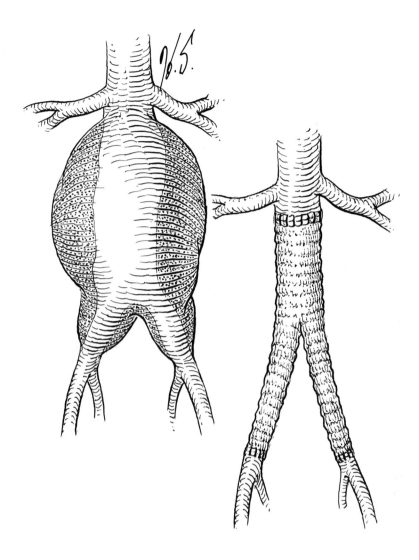

Figure 94. Abdominal aortic aneurysm (left) treated by
excision and replacement with a Dacron graft (right)

Aneurysm of the Descending Thoracic Aorta

Aneurysms of the descending thoracic aorta are usually fusiform and
arteriosclerotic in origin. They are most common in men and may occur at
any age, but most frequently develop between the ages of fifty and eighty.
Symptoms may not be present, but when they do occur they usually relate to
the compression of surrounding structures, producing pain in the chest or
back which may radiate to the neck, shoulders or abdomen. When the
aneurysm compresses the trachea, it may cause a hacking cough. Increasing

pain is an ominous sign of progressive enlargement and impending rupture. Precise diagnosis is made by aortography.

Surgical treatment is suggested except when conditions such as severe

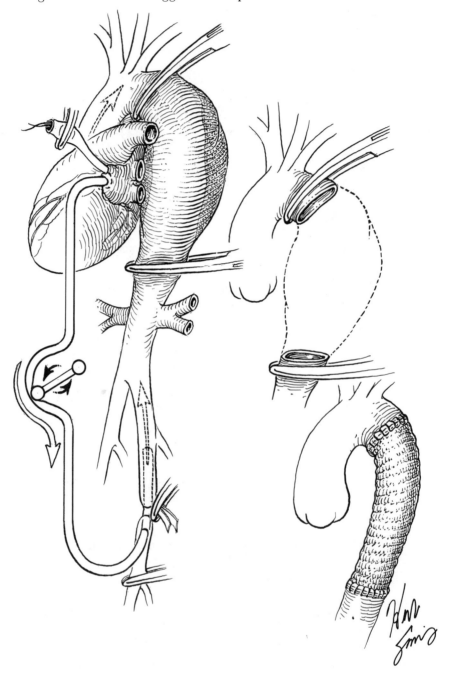

Figure 95. Surgical technique for the treatment of an aneurysm of the descending thoracic aorta

debilitating disease or heart failure are present. The operation is performed by entering the left side of the chest through an incision between the ribs. The aneurysm is excised between occluding clamps on the aorta and replaced with a Dacron graft (Figure 95).

Results of the operation are excellent, with an operative risk between 5 and 10 percent. There is a small (2 to 4 percent) incidence of paraplegia secondary to lack of blood supply to the spinal cord following the operation. Although various methods have been used to prevent this occurrence, none have proved completely effective.

Aneurysms of the Ascending Aorta

These aneurysms may occur at any age, even during the first ten years of life when they are usually of congenital origin. Most occur between the ages of forty and eighty, and are of arteriosclerotic origin. Some are of undetermined etiology and resemble aneurysms of the sinus of valsalva, especially in younger patients. Others may be associated with aortic valve insufficiency. Symptoms may or may not be present, and the condition most often is discovered during a routine physical examination or chest x-ray. Pain in the chest is one of the most common symptoms and if aortic valve insufficiency is present, early heart failure may occur. Precise diagnosis is made by aortography.

Surgical treatment is recommended in all patients except when there is severe associated disease that would make the risk prohibitive. The operation is performed using the heart-lung machine and consists of excising the aneurysmal segment and replacing it with a Dacron graft (Figure 96). If aortic valve insufficiency is present, an artificial valve is used to replace the diseased one. Results of this operation are excellent, with a risk of about 5 to 10 percent.

Aneurysm of the Aortic Arch

This is one of the most serious and difficult forms of aortic aneurysm to treat because it involves the major arteries supplying blood to the brain. It occurs predominantly in males between the ages of fifty and seventy. Symptoms are produced by compression of surrounding structures, particularly the trachea and esophagus. Pain in the chest or at the base of the neck is common, and other symptoms may be a hacking cough or difficulty in swallowing. The precise diagnosis is made by aortography.

Surgery is recommended unless there is associated disease that would create a prohibitive risk. The procedure is performed using the heart-lung machine with connections to the arteries supplying blood to the brain and the coronary arteries (Figure 97). Occluding clamps are placed on the aorta distal to the aneurysm and on the major arteries arising from the aortic arch.

The aneurysm is then excised and replaced by a Dacron graft with connections to the arteries normally arising from the aortic arch. Results of this operation are excellent, with an operative risk of about 10 to 15 percent.

Thoracoabdominal Aneurysm

These aneurysms are fusiform in nature and usually occur in the lower descending thoracic aorta with extension into the abdominal aorta for varying distances. They occur most frequently in men between the ages of fifty and seventy. Symptoms are similar to those associated with aneurysm of

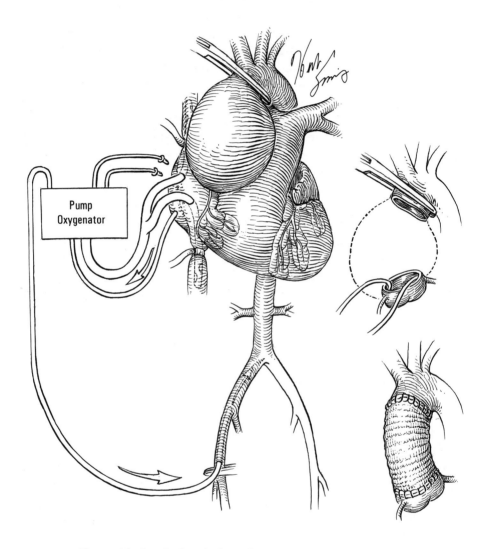

Figure 96. Surgical technique for the treatment of an aneurysm of the ascending thoracic aorta

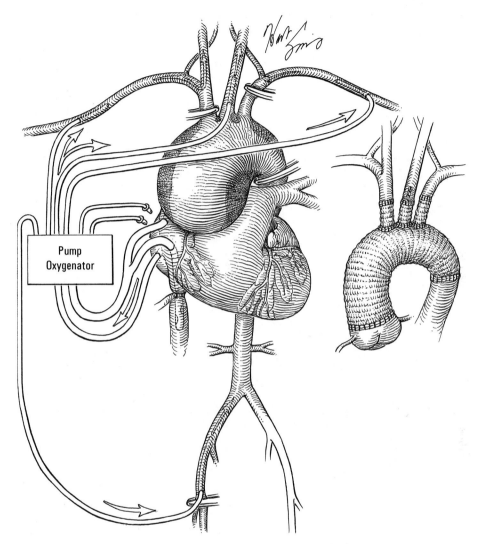

Figure 97. Surgical technique for the treatment of an aneurysm involving the entire aortic arch

the abdominal aorta, except that pain may occur higher in the abdomen and the chest or back. Aortography is essential for precise diagnosis.

A special technique has been developed for this type of aneurysm. First a Dacron bypass graft is attached from the descending thoracic aorta to the abdominal aorta or iliac arteries beyond the aneurysm (Figure 98). Additional side grafts are attached from this main graft to the renal arteries, superior mesenteric artery and celiac axis. The aneurysm then is excised and the two ends of the aorta are closed by suture. Results of the operation are excellent, with an operative risk of about 15 percent.

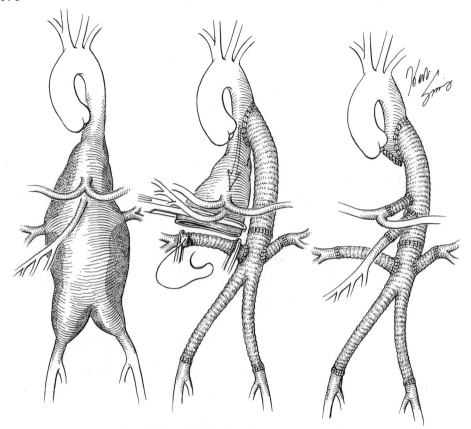

Figure 98. Surgical technique for the treatment of an aneurysm involving the thoracoabdominal aorta

Dissecting Aneurysms of the Aorta

This is one of the most serious and grave forms of aneurysmal disease. Death results within a few weeks in over half of the patients and within a year in 90 percent. It occurs predominantly in men between forty and seventy years of age. Half the patients have severe hypertension. Symptoms usually develop with a sudden onset of pain in the chest radiating to the back, shoulders, neck, abdomen or legs. The condition is sometimes confused with an acute heart attack. A "marching" nature of the pain is common, as it radiates upward or downward. Transitory numbness in the face or extremities and even paraplegia may occur.

The basic lesion of dissecting aneurysms seems to be a degeneration of the media of the aorta, not related to arteriosclerosis. It is sometimes associated with a condition known as *Marfan's syndrome*. A tear in the intimal layer allows blood to enter the diseased media and the force of blood pressure with each heart beat develops a separation between these layers. This dissecting process occurs in only a part of the circumference of the aorta but, depending on the type of separation, may extend throughout the aorta and even into the arteries of the legs.

There are three types of dissecting aneurysms (Figure 99). In Type I, the dissecting process extends throughout the aorta and sometimes beyond the

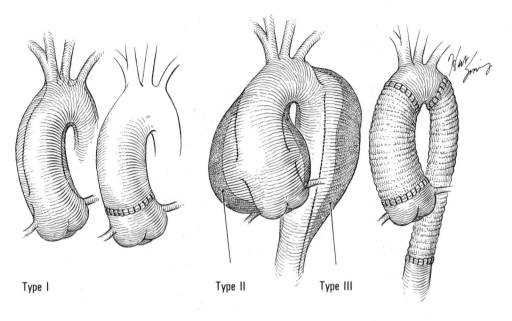

Type I   Type II   Type III

Figure 99. Surgical technique for the treatment of the three types of dissecting aortic aneurysms

bifurcation of the abdominal aorta; Type II is similar but is limited to the ascending aorta, with aortic valve insufficiency usually present. In Type III, the dissecting process begins in the upper portion of the descending thoracic aorta and extends downward for varying distances, sometimes even into the abdominal aorta. The precise diagnosis and type of dissecting aneurysm is determined by aortography.

Surgical treatment depends upon the type of dissection and the condition of the patient. In the case of Type I, it is preferable to first employ medical measures in an effort to stabilize the process and to reduce the level of blood pressure. Surgery is suggested if there is a progression of the disease indicating possible impending rupture. With the patient on the heart-lung machine, the diseased segment of the ascending aorta is resected and replaced with a Dacron graft (Figure 99).

Surgical treatment is suggested in most cases of Type II dissecting aneurysm soon after diagnosis. The procedure uses the heart-lung machine and is similar to that described for aneurysms of the ascending aorta; often an artificial aortic valve is used to replace the incompetent one.

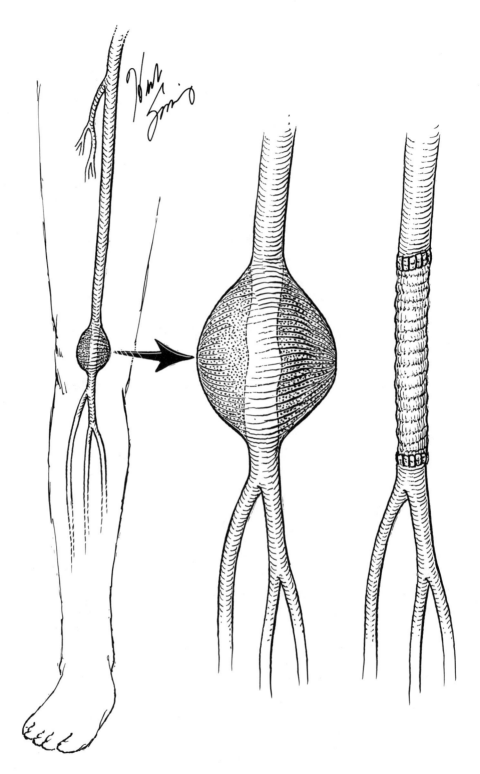

Figure 100. Surgical technique for the repair of an aneurysm of the popliteal artery in the leg

Surgical treatment also is recommended in the majority of patients with Type III aneurysms as soon as the diagnosis is made. The operation involves resection and Dacron graft replacement similar to that used for fusiform aneurysms of the descending thoracic aorta. When the dissecting process extends into the abdominal aorta, the two walls of the false lumen are reapproximated by suture before attaching the graft to the distal end of the aorta.

Results of these operations are excellent, with an overall risk of approximately 12 percent. The highest risk is with the Type I aneurysm, which has a mortality of about 30 percent. Long-term results are excellent, with some patients surviving twenty years or more after surgery.

Aneurysm of Major Peripheral Arteries

These aneurysms are usually localized and fusiform in nature. They most frequently involve the femoral, popliteal, carotid and subclavian arteries. They may occur in the major arteries to the abdominal viscera such as the renal, superior mesenteric, celiac and splenic arteries. They are found most often in men between fifty and seventy years of age. Surgical treatment is suggested for most of these aneurysms and consists of resection and Dacron graft replacement (Figure 100). Results are excellent, with a very low risk of about one percent or less.

13

ACQUIRED HEART DISEASES AFFECTING THE PERICARDIUM, MYOCARDIUM AND VALVES

*I*N contrast to congenital heart disease, acquired heart disease is caused by conditions which occur after birth; atherosclerosis and coronary artery disease are typical examples. This chapter is devoted to acquired heart disease other than that affecting the coronary arteries. These diseases may affect the pericardium, which is the covering of the heart; the myocardium itself; or the valves of the heart and their associated structures.

Pericarditis

Inflammation of the pericardial sac may be acute or chronic in nature. Acute pericarditis is associated with an accumulation of fluid in the pericardial cavity around the heart. If the condition persists, or is associated

178

with subsequent deposition of fibrotic tissue, it becomes a long-term illness referred to as chronic pericarditis. Acute pericarditis may occur as a complication of a myocardial infarction or cardiac surgery; it can be secondary to a viral or bacterial infection or to a metabolic disturbance such as uremia, which occurs in kidney failure. Acute pericarditis usually does not interfere with the functioning of the heart, but may cause severe pain. It usually accompanies an acute illness with fever and chills. On listening to the heartbeat with a stethoscope, a "rub" may be heard due to friction between the pericardial sac and the epicardial surface of the heart during systole and diastole. In chronic pericarditis, a constriction may interfere with the flow of blood, producing back pressure. Fluid may also accumulate in the lower extremities and congestion of the liver may occur. This condition is referred to as right-sided heart failure.

The treatment of pericarditis depends upon the cause. The most common infectious cause of chronic pericarditis is tuberculosis. If a bacterial agent is the cause, antibiotic treatment and bed rest are indicated. Pericarditis associated with a myocardial infarction or after heart surgery may require only bed rest and control of the fever and pain. But chronic constrictive pericarditis may call for more than treatment of the heart failure with medication. Stripping off a section of the pericardial covering by a procedure called a pericardiectomy can relieve the back pressure on the right side of the heart as well as many other symptoms.

Myocardial Disease

While coronary artery disease may result in damage to the myocardium, it is not primarily a disease of the myocardial muscle itself. The term "myocardial disease" describes a heterogeneous collection of disorders which include inflammatory processes, called myocarditis; infiltrative processes in which the myocardium becomes filled with substances such as amyloid; and fibrotic diseases in which the heart muscle is replaced by fibrous connective tissue. Various infectious agents may cause myocarditis. Dysfunction of the heart muscle can result in a condition called *cardiomyopathy*. This is a syndrome or a group of diseases in which the heart is enlarged and failing, and the heart muscle is not functioning adequately. If an underlying cause is identifiable, the cardiomyopathy is said to be secondary and treatment depends upon the cause. Agents such as alcohol may cause cardiomyopathy in susceptible patients. If no underlying cause can be detected, then the cardiomyopathy is called primary. If an underlying cause is identified, then it should be directly treated. An effort should be made to control associated heart failure and arrhythmias. Primary cardiomyopathy may require long periods of bed rest and there is no satisfactory or generally accepted treatment at the present time.

Acute Rheumatic Fever and Rheumatic Heart Disease

A streptococcal organism is the cause of rheumatic fever. Acute attacks of rheumatic fever occur most commonly in children between seven and fourteen years of age during the winter months, and the disease is associated with low socio-economic conditions. The advent of penicillin, which provides an effective treatment for this variety of streptococcal infection, greatly reduced the incidence of rheumatic fever and its complications in the United States. An attack of acute rheumatic fever usually begins two or three weeks after the infection of the throat or tonsils. There is not always a history of a previous sore throat, however. Rheumatic fever is thought to be a hypersensitive reaction to the beta-streptococcal organism. In this sense, rheumatic fever represents a type of allergic reaction to the beta-streptococcus. The most frequent manifestation is an inflammation of the large joints of the body, called migratory polyarthritis, which occurs in approximately 85 percent of all cases. Inflammation of the heart is seen about 65 percent of the time, and may be manifested by increased heart rate, first-degree heart block, the presence of a murmur, and a friction rub over the heart due to pericarditis. About 30 percent of all patients develop a condition called chorea, or St. Vitus dance, which is a disorder of the central nervous system. It may even occur without any of the other clinical features of rheumatic fever. Chorea is characterized by spastic twitchings of the muscles and occurs most commonly in prepubertal females. Thus, during an attack of acute rheumatic fever, there may be inflammation of the joints, the pericardium, the myocardium and the heart valves.

Proper early diagnosis and antibiotic treatment with penicillin during the acute attacks are of the utmost importance in order to eradicate the streptococcal organism from the nose and throat. Bed rest and aspirin also help to relieve the pain in the joints. During the acute phase of the disease, the valves of the heart may become inflamed and filled with edema fluid. A pathological lesion, characteristic of rheumatic fever, is seen through the microscope on the endocardial, or interior, surface of the heart. Called the Aschoff nodule, it is a collection of several types of cells around a center of dead tissue. A long period of recovery is required following rheumatic fever. Once the acute phase has occurred, penicillin has relatively little effect on the course of the illness.

Rheumatic heart disease occurs years after acute rheumatic fever, and although it usually affects the mitral and aortic valves, it can also result in damage to the tricuspid valve. It is important to distinguish whether valve damage is caused by bacterial endocarditis or rheumatic heart disease. In bacterial endocarditis, the damage to the heart valve is actually a result of a bacterial infection on the valve itself. By contrast, in rheumatic heart disease the major damage to the valve does not occur at the time of the acute infection. Once an individual has had an attack of acute rheumatic fever, the heart valves may sustain severe damage from further attacks. In such individuals, it is imperative to maintain future prophylaxis with antibiotics to prevent further beta-streptococcal infections and recurrence of rheumatic fever.

Endocarditis

Endocarditis is a condition in which the endocardium of the heart is inflamed. Usually this condition is caused by a bacteria which affects the valves. Often a heart valve previously damaged by rheumatic heart disease or damaged from birth will be the site affected by bacterial endocarditis. The disease may be classified as acute and subacute. The acute type usually arises as a complication of severe bacterial infection of the bloodstream called septicemia. A patient with acute bacterial endocarditis is extremely ill with fever and chills. The heartbeat is very rapid and congestive heart failure may occur. Arterial emboli are sometimes released from the damaged heart valves. The valves themselves may be practically destroyed in a relatively short period of time. An infected embolus may lodge in an artery and produce a type of aneurysm called a *mycotic* aneurysm. Successful treatment requires identification of the infectious organism and an immediate and vigorous program of appropriate antibiotics.

Subacute bacterial endocarditis often is caused by organisms found in the upper respiratory and gastrointestinal tracts, such as the Streptococcus viridans and the enterococci, which are noninfectious under ordinary circumstances. A heart valve damaged from rheumatic heart disease or a congenital defect is more susceptible to attack by this insidious disease than a normal valve. An attack may follow oral surgery or dental work in which bacteria get into the bloodstream. Whereas acute bacterial endocarditis results in large deposits forming on the surface of the heart valves, the subacute type produces smaller deposits. Damage to the valve may occur with either variety of the disease. Treatment for both acute and subacute bacterial endocarditis is aimed at identifying the causative agent and effectively treating it with antibiotics. Intravenous antibiotic treatment is often administered, sometimes for prolonged periods of time. Prophylactic steps should be subsequently taken, such as the use of antibiotics at the time dental work is to be done.

Mitral Valve Disease

Damage to the mitral valve produces progressive thickening and loss of pliability of the valve leaflets with fusion of the edges, contraction of the *chorda tendineae* and *calcium deposition* (Figure 101). These changes may produce a narrowing of the valve opening, called mitral stenosis, in which there is obstruction to blood flow between the left atrium and left ventricle. Alternatively, there may be incompetence of the valve, i.e. an inability of the valve leaflets to close, called mitral insufficiency. Although either stenosis or

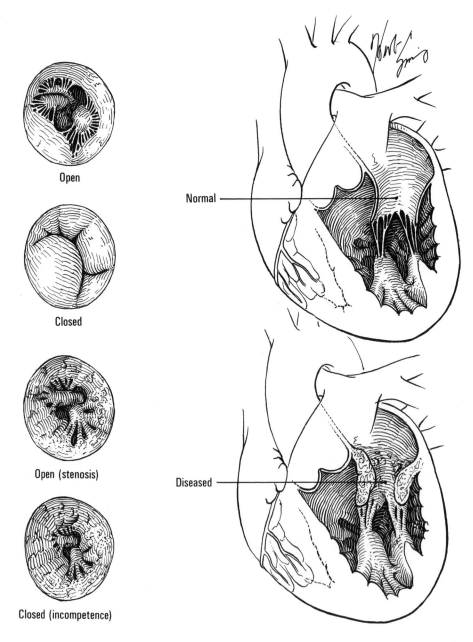

Open

Closed

Open (stenosis)

Closed (incompetence)

Normal

Diseased

Figure 101. A diseased mitral valve (below) compared to a normal mitral valve (above)

incompetence of the valve is the predominant dysfunction, there often is an element of both. When narrowing of the valve is the major change, the pressure in the left atrium increases, producing an elevation in pulmonary venous pressure. This increases the work of the right ventricle and ultimately

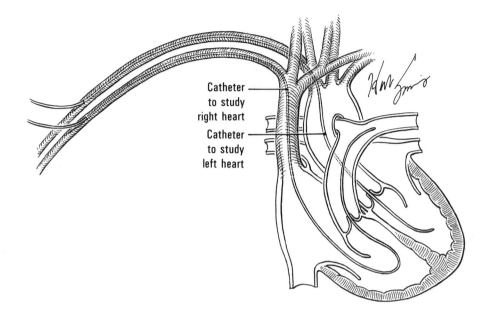

Catheter to study right heart

Catheter to study left heart

Figure 102. Catheters are passed into the left and right side of the heart to obtain the information necessary for precise diagnosis of valvular disease.

results in heart failure. Along with this sequence of events, *atrial fibrillation* may produce irregular, poor contractions of the left atrium. Irregular contraction of the left ventricle may develop, further aggravating the problem. When the predominant valve dysfunction is incompetence, blood is shunted back and forth between the left atrium and left ventricle *(mitral regurgitation)*, thus increasing the work load on the heart, and ultimately resulting in pulmonary congestion and heart failure. The disease occurs about four times more frequently in women than in men.

The effect upon heart function varies with the degree of pathological change in the mitral valve. In mild forms of the disease, the heart may compensate adequately and the patient may have little disability. Most patients, however, suffer gradual and progressive disability over a period of years. Studies of the natural history of the uncorrected disease have shown that about one in five patients with mitral stenosis will die within one year after first seeking help of a physician; three out of five patients will die within ten years.

Treatment of mitral valve disease may be medical or surgical, depending upon the degree of disability. Surgery is suggested for patients who have symptoms of early heart failure and dysfunction, and for those who develop certain complications such as *peripheral embolization* from a clot in the left atrium. More precise information concerning the need for surgical treatment may be determined by special laboratory tests such as cardiac catherization (Figure 102).

Operations for mitral valve disease either repair or replace the valve, depending upon the extent of the damage. In certain types of mitral regurgitation in which the valve leaflets are not significantly damaged, repair may be possible. In pure mitral stenosis in which the valve leaflets are not badly damaged and are still pliable, it may be possible to repair the valve by separating or dividing the fused edges. Prior to the development of the heart-lung machine this was done by a "closed" technique. The index finger was inserted through an opening in the left atrium, or an instrument was inserted through the left ventricle, to dilate the valve opening. Many surgeons now prefer to use an "open" technique in which use of the heart-lung machine allows the heart to be opened through an incision in the left atrium to permit direct vision of the mitral valve. This enables a more accurate assessment of the damage and a more precise technique for dividing or separating the fused edges of the valve. Moreover, in some cases it may not be possible to open the narrowed valve adequately without inducing incompetence. Under these circumstances valve replacement may be necessary and can be performed immediately.

In our experience, surgical treatment for most patients with severe mitral stenosis and mitral regurgitation requires replacement of the valve. Most heart centers today use an artificial valve, although a few surgeons prefer to use a *homograft valve* (one taken from a cadaver) or a *heterograft valve* (one taken from an animal such as a pig). A number of different types of artificial valves have been developed for this purpose, most of which use the *ball valve principle* (Figure 103). The ball itself, however, may be in the form of a disc, especially when designed for mitral or tricuspid valve replacement. In this type of valve, the ball or disc is enclosed in a cage consisting of three or four wired struts with an opening at the bottom somewhat smaller than the ball, so that the opening is closed when the ball is seated on it. With an increase in pressure on the inflow side of this opening, the ball moves into the cage allowing blood to flow around it. With the drop in pressure that occurs in the next phase of the heart's cycle, the ball drops back against the seat of the opening, preventing blood from flowing back.

In recent years, great improvements have been made in these artificial valves and most of them now provide good results. Through our own research, we have developed a valve that uses a material called pyrolytic carbon for the ball or disc and for the seat of the valve (Figure 104). Dacron velour is used for the sewing ring. Over the past ten years, this type of valve has proved to be highly satisfactory.

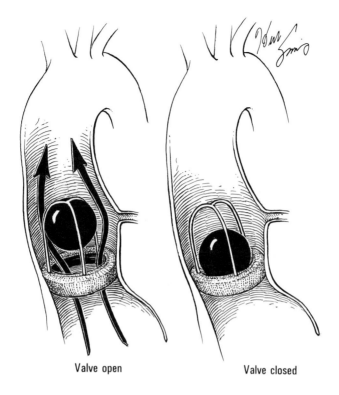

Valve open   Valve closed

Figure 103. The function of a prosthetic ball valve

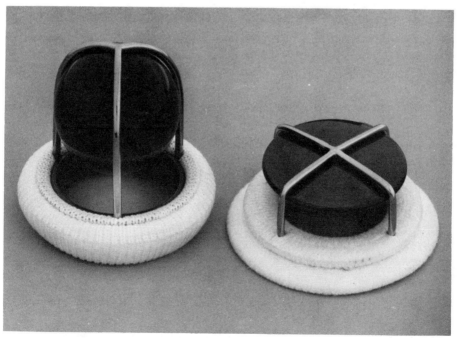

Figure 104. The DeBakey pyrolytic carbon prosthetic valves

The operation is performed by exposing the heart through a vertical incision in the breastbone or through a diagonal incision between the ribs and across the breastbone. After placing the patient on the heart-lung machine, the mitral valve is exposed through an opening in the left atrium (Figure 105). The damaged valve is then excised and sutures are placed circumferentially through the natural valve annulus and then passed through the sewing ring of the artificial valve. The prosthetic valve then is seated into the annulus and the sutures are tied to firmly attach the prosthesis to the annulus. Heart function is restored after removing all air from the heart chambers and closing the incision in the left atrium. The operative risk is now no more than 10 or 15 percent, and in patients without severe long-term heart failure it is less than 5 percent. Most patients recover and resume relatively normal activities.

Aortic Valve Disease

Damage to the aortic valve may result in narrowing of the opening caused by thickening, distortion and fusion of the valve cusps, as well as by *calcification* (Figure 106). Sometimes damage to the aortic valve results in valve incompetence. In stenosis there is obstruction of the flow of blood from the left ventricle, which increases the total work required of the heart, thereby causing progressive hypertrophy and failure as well as arrhythmia.

Ultimately, patients develop symptoms of heart failure, with attacks of shortness of breath, chest pain and syncope, or temporary loss of consciousness. These signs often are a prelude to death. In about one-fifth of the patients, sudden death occurs without preexisting symptoms, which is believed to be due to arrhythmia. Associated coronary artery disease is not uncommon.

Although rheumatic fever is the most common cause of aortic insufficiency, it may also be caused by destruction of the valve leaflets by bacterial infection, by certain lesions of the ascending aorta such as syphilis, by dissecting aneurysms, by dilatation of the annulus and, occasionally, by severe trauma. As a consequence of the valve incompetence, blood flowing out of the left ventricle during systole is partially regurgitated back into the ventricle during diastole. This produces an increased work load on the heart, causing it to enlarge and ultimately fail. Once symptoms of shortness of breath or pain in the chest develop, the prognosis is very poor and life expectancy is reduced to possibly one to three years.

Surgical treatment is suggested for all patients who develop symptoms, as well as for those without symptoms whose examinations suggest progressive disease and a strain developing on the left ventricle. These determinations are best made by studies which include cardiac catherization. Surgical treatment should not be delayed until the patient develops severe symptoms. The operation consists of excision of the diseased aortic valve and replacement. Most surgeons prefer an artificial valve over a homograft. The type of valve we have used for about ten years is the pyrolytic carbon ball valve described earlier (Figure 104). Our experience with this valve in over a thousand cases has been highly gratifying.

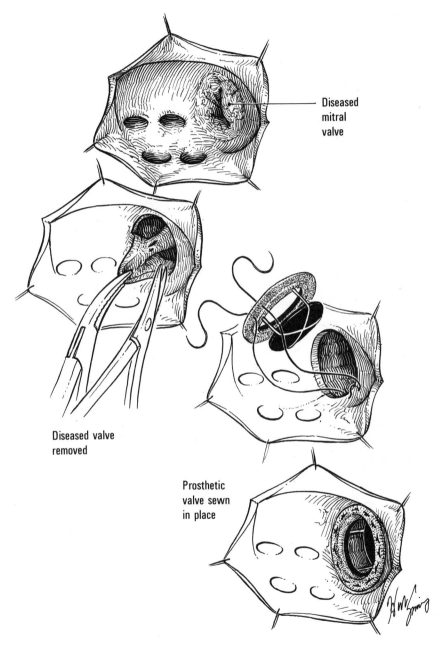

Figure 105. Surgical technique for the replacement of a diseased mitral valve

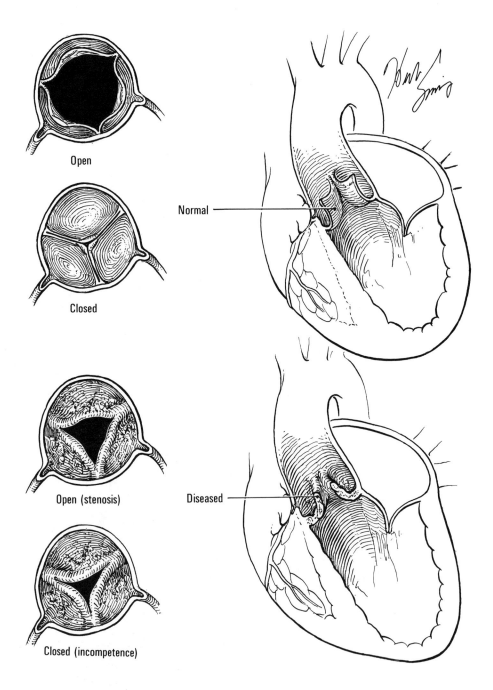

Open

Closed

Normal

Open (stenosis)

Closed (incompetence)

Diseased

Figure 106. A diseased aortic valve (below) compared to a
normal aortic valve (above)

The operative procedure exposes the heart through a vertical incision in
the breastbone. The patient is placed on the heart-lung machine and the
ascending aorta is occluded (Figure 107). The valve is then exposed by an
incision in the aorta. After excising the diseased valve, the sutures are placed

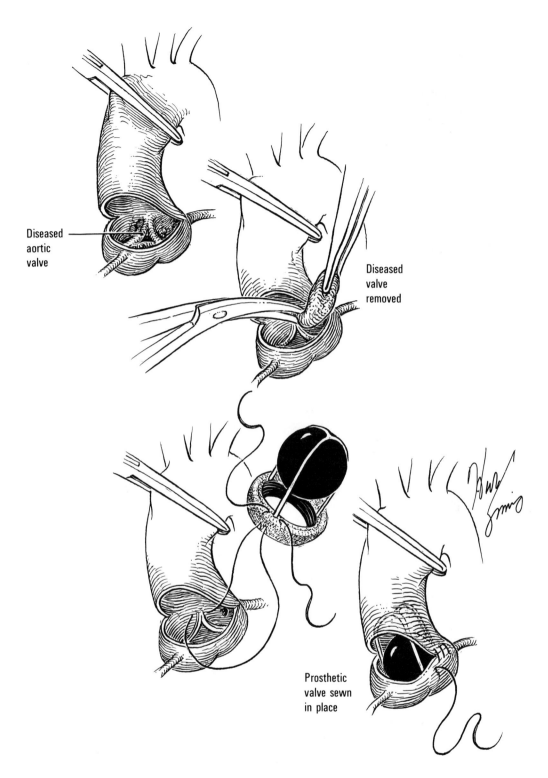

Diseased aortic valve

Diseased valve removed

Prosthetic valve sewn in place

Figure 107. The surgical technique for replacement of a diseased aortic valve with a prosthesis

around the remaining annulus and then through the sewing ring of the ball valve. The valve is seated into the annulus and firmly attached by tying the sutures. Air in the heart is removed, the incision in the aorta is closed, and heart function is restored.

Results following aortic valve replacement are excellent, and the operative risk is often less than 5 percent. Long-term results are very good, with most patients resuming relatively normal lives.

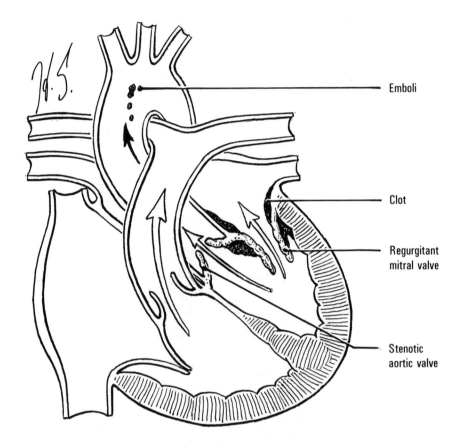

Figure 108. Disease in both the aortic and mitral valves. Clot forming around the base of the mitral valve and in the left atrium may break off and form emboli that pass out the aorta to lodge in an artery in another part of the body.

Combined Valvular Disease

In some patients there is significant disease of both the mitral valve and the aortic valve (Figure 108). Under these circumstances it may be necessary to replace both valves. This is done in the same manner as described for each valve separately. The risk of this combined procedure is about 10 percent and the results are very satisfactory.

In a small proportion of patients there may be significant damage of the tricuspid valve in association with mitral valve disease or with mitral and aortic valve disease. Occasionally it may be necessary to replace all three valves (Figure 109).

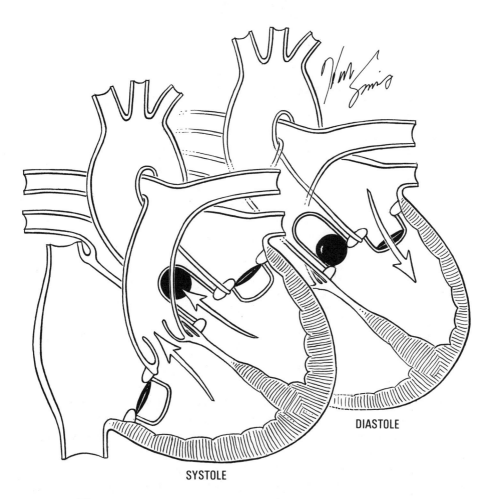

DIASTOLE

SYSTOLE

Figure 109. Diagram of heart function when all three valves are replaced with prostheses

14

HYPERTENSION

*A*N elevation of arterial blood pressure is called hypertension. In recent years hypertension has been referred to as "the silent killer" because it often produces no noticeable symptoms before severe damage occurs in the heart, cardiovascular system and other organs. Hypertension may result in an early stroke, cause enlargement of the heart, damage the kidneys and cause them to fail, lead to the formation of aneurysms and rupture of the large arteries, and may result in damage to the retina (Figure 110).

A systolic blood pressure of 140 millimeters of mercury or over and a diastolic pressure of 90 millimeters or over are usually used to define hypertension. Life insurance companies consider blood pressure to be the single most important factor in determining an individual's longevity. Life insurance statistics leave little doubt that there is a strong correlation between the blood pressure and the risk of death. For both men and women in the United States, systolic and diastolic pressures gradually rise with age. Among certain primitive populations where there is essentially no hypertension, blood pressure does not rise with age. According to data from the

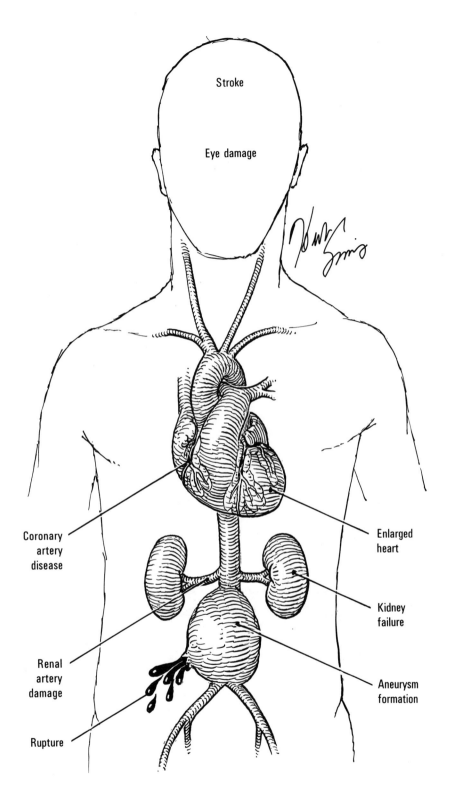

Stroke

Eye damage

Coronary
artery
disease

Enlarged
heart

Kidney
failure

Renal
artery
damage

Aneurysm
formation

Rupture

Figure 110. The consequences of hypertension

Metropolitan Life Insurance Company, the life expectancy for a thirty-five-year-old man is reduced by approximately sixteen years if he has a blood pressure over 150/100 as compared to a normal reading of 120/80. For a forty-five-year-old man, the reduction in life expectancy is twelve years with such a high reading and about eight or nine years for a woman.

According to the data supplied by the American Heart Association, there are more than 25 million hypertensives in the United States. The frequency of untreated hypertension is one of the saddest commentaries on our health care system today. The disease is about twice as common in blacks as in whites, perhaps affecting one out of four adult blacks. Only about half of the 25 million hypertensives are aware of their problem, and out of this group, only about one-half are under treatment. Many are not being treated effectively—perhaps only about 10 percent are under adequate control. Hypertension per se is listed as the primary cause of death for about 60,000 people each year in the United States. In addition, it is the major risk factor for stroke, and one of three major risk factors for heart attacks and coronary artery disease. About 200,000 Americans die of strokes and more than 600,000 are cut down by heart attacks each year. A hypertensive individual who is not receiving treatment has four times the risk of having a stroke as an individual with normal blood pressure.

The blood pressure depends upon cardiac output and the resistance to blood flow through the peripheral arteries. For many years, it was thought that older patients with atherosclerosis required a higher blood pressure in order to force the blood through damaged vessels. About forty-five years ago, Dr. Samuel Levine in Boston observed a very high incidence of hypertension in patients with myocardial infarctions and associated the two phenomena.

Despite much work on the physiological regulation of the blood pressure, the mechanisms involved are still not completely understood. There are small signal receivers in the walls of arteries called *baroreceptors* which are sensitive to changes in blood pressure and are found in strategic locations such as the carotid sinus and aortic arch (Figure 111). If the blood pressure goes up, the baroreceptors send signals through the nerves to relax the arterioles and slow the heart, thereby returning blood pressure to normal. The blood pressure changes during the day to meet the demands of various situations. During times of fright, the blood pressure rises, while during times of rest, relaxation and sleep, it decreases.

In addition to the minute-by-minute regulation of the blood pressure by the nervous system, the fluids and salts retained and excreted by the kidneys are extremely important determinants of the arterial pressure. Excessive retention of fluid and salt can lead to an elevation of blood pressure. Fluid and sodium excretion by the kidneys is regulated by hormones. A hormone called aldosterone, produced by the adrenal cortex, causes a retention of sodium and a loss of potassium by the kidney; therefore, its overproduction can cause hypertension. A peptide substance called renin is produced by the kidney and released when there is a fall in the blood pressure and blood flow to the kidney. Renin is converted to another peptide called angiotesion II, which causes an increase in secretion of aldosterone and a constriction of arterioles (Figure 111). A low salt diet is one of the ways to treat

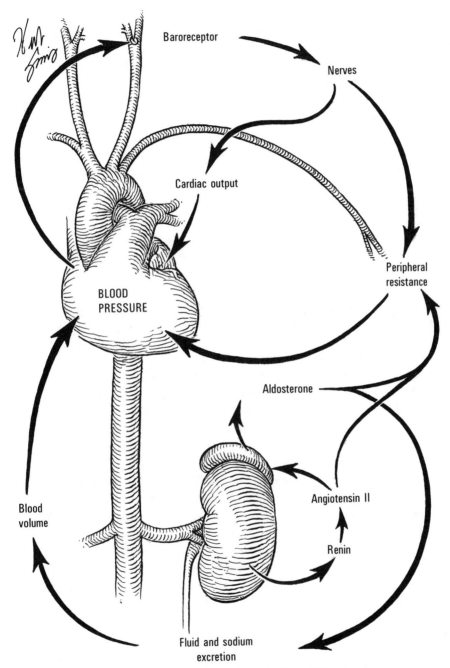

Figure 111. The mechanism of regulation of blood pressure

hypertension. The use of diuretic agents also helps to promote the excretion of fluid and sodium by the kidneys.

Doctor John Laragh of New York City has suggested that many hypertensive subjects fall into one of two categories. One group overproduces renin, while the second group has low levels of renin. According to Dr. Laragh, the group with a high renin secretion runs a high risk of developing cardiovascular complications, while the low renin subjects have a relatively low risk. Dr. Laragh suggests that patients with high renin levels be treated with drugs, such as propanolol, which block the arteriolar constriction. The low renin subjects would be given diuretics to increase their water excretion. Further study will be necessary to determine the significance of high versus low renin in a hypertensive.

Another renal system that may regulate blood pressure by influencing salt and fluid excretion is the kallikrein-kinin sequence. Renal kallikrein causes the release of the kinin substances from the kidney. These substances increase the loss of fluid and/or sodium by the kidney. Some studies have suggested that there is a deficiency of renal kallikrein in hypertension, which would promote sodium and water retention.

Types of Hypertension: Curable Versus Treatable

Reference has already been made to two types of hypertension: that caused by low renin and that caused by high renin concentrations. One of the most common ways of referring to hypertension is benign versus malignant. This is misleading because it implies that nonmalignant hypertension is not serious. This impression is wrong and the term benign hypertension probably should be discarded altogether. Malignant hypertension refers to an accelerated form of the disease in which the kidneys and central nervous system are affected. It is rapidly fatal unless brought under control with medication. The introduction of drugs to lower blood pressure has been a significant development in the past twenty years and has decreased the mortality from accelerated hypertension.

The discovery of an elevation of systolic or diastolic blood pressure, or both, requires medical attention. The physical and emotional condition of the individual and the clinical findings must be considered, since under certain circumstances, an increase in blood pressure is a normal physiological response. For example, racing car drivers and individuals with other hazardous occupations may raise their blood pressure to hypertensive levels at times of acute physical or emotional stress. The blood pressure should return to normal, however, when the stress is removed.

There are a number of medical causes of elevated blood pressure, which may be considered curable because an underlying removable cause can be identified (Figure 112). When such curable causes are excluded, we are then left with a heterogeneous collection of noncurable varieties which we call

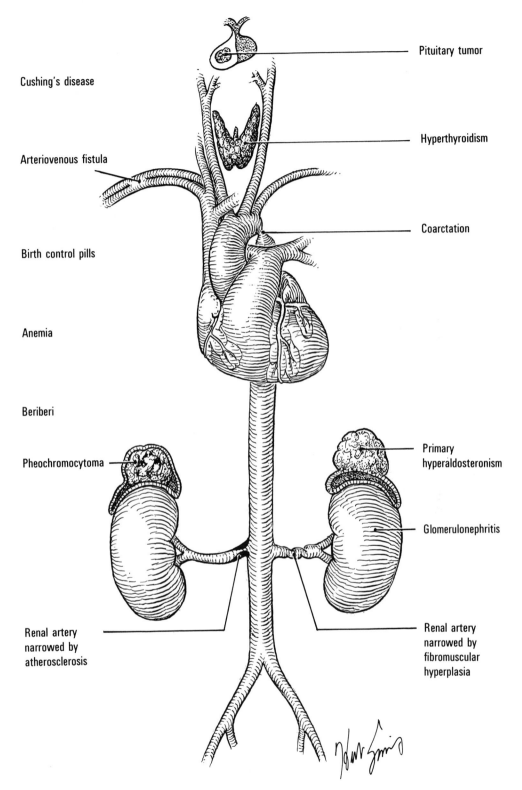

Cushing's disease

Pituitary tumor

Arteriovenous fistula

Hyperthyroidism

Birth control pills

Coarctation

Anemia

Beriberi

Pheochromocytoma

Primary
hyperaldosteronism

Glomerulonephritis

Renal artery
narrowed by
atherosclerosis

Renal artery
narrowed by
fibromuscular
hyperplasia

Figure 112. The curable causes of hypertension

essential hypertension. The majority of individuals with hypertension, as much as 85 percent today, fall into this category. The more we learn about blood pressure, its regulation and the factors that can upset its control, the smaller the group of patients becomes whose hypertension is called essential.

For example, let us take a patient who comes to a doctor's office for a checkup. Let us say that both systolic and diastolic pressure are found to be elevated. What possible causes might the physician uncover by proceeding with a medical workup? One curable cause is occlusive disease, affecting one or both renal arteries (Figure 112). Narrowing of the renal artery to the kidney may be caused by atherosclerosis or by another disease process called fibromuscular hyperplasia. Let us suppose there is an atherosclerotic plaque obstructing the artery to one of the two kidneys. The urinalysis and blood tests of kidney function may show no abnormality until relatively advanced disease is present. The physiological effect of a blockage in the renal artery is to diminish the blood flow to the affected kidney. This abnormality may in some instances be diagnosed by an x-ray test in which a radiopaque dye is injected into a vein. The x-ray may show that the affected kidney has a decrease in the rate at which the dye is excreted. In order to pinpoint the site of the blockage, an arteriogram may be performed. In this test the radiopaque dye is injected into the artery to delineate the precise site and extent of the blockage. Another diagnostic test measures the concentration of renin in each renal vein. As discussed earlier, the kidney responds to a decrease in blood flow by releasing an increased amount of renin. Thus, the concentration of renin will be higher in the vein from the affected kidney than in that from the normal one. Surgical treatment of the diseased renal artery by bypassing the narrowed area may cure the hypertension. Thus, renal artery stenosis represents a classical form of curable hypertension.

Hypertension may also be caused by a small tumor of the adrenal cortex where aldosterone is produced (Figure 112). The resulting condition is called primary hyperaldosteronism. In this condition, the level of circulating aldosterone is increased, the level of renin is lowered, and the concentration of serum sodium is usually increased relative to that of potassium. All of these effects are caused by the increased level of circulating aldosterone. The increased concentration of the hormone leads to sodium and fluid retention, thus resulting in hypertension. The treatment is surgical removal of the adrenal tumor. Another type of adrenal tumor that can cause hypertension is called a pheochromocytoma. This type of tumor originates in the medulla of the adrenal gland where the adrenal hormones, adrenalin and noradrenalin are produced. Their net effect is to increase the heart rate and the strength of the contractions of the heart. Noradrenalin can cause constriction of small, muscular arteries and arterioles which leads to an increase in peripheral resistance to blood flow. When a pheochromocytoma is present, it may be possible to demonstrate the presence of increased quantities of breakdown products of the adrenal hormones in the urine. Again, the treatment is surgical, which may be by removal of the pheochromocytoma.

A surgically curable cause of hypertension, often detected in childhood, is a narrowing of the aorta, referred to as a coarctation (see Chapter 7).

Hypertension, caused by an excessive accumulation of fluid and salt, complicates a disease called glomerulonephritis, which is an inflammation of the kidney. Provided that the kidneys do not sustain permanent damage, this type of hypertension disappears after the disease runs its course. Other curable causes of hypertension include Cushing's disease, in which there is an overproduction of the adrenal cortical hormones other than aldosterone; the presence of a brain tumor, expecially one of the pituitary gland; and the use of birth control pills in certain women (Figure 112).

Systemic hypertension with normal diastolic blood pressure also occurs in curable conditions associated with a high cardiac output, such as anemia, hyperthyroidism, beriberi, heart disease, and arterio-venous fistula. When the curable causes of hypertension have been ruled out, we are left with the diagnosis of essential hypertension. A treatable rather than curable situation in which there is an elevation of the systolic blood pressure without a significant rise in the diastolic blood pressure exists in elderly individuals whose arteries are less distensible because of calcification and arteriosclerosis.

There is not uniform agreement as to when hypertension requires treatment. From a study recently carried out in the Veterans Administration hospitals in the United States, there seems little doubt that treatment of blood pressure greater than a diastolic reading of 105 millimeters of mercury can lead to a decrease in death and disability from stroke. Treatment must be individualized but it generally is recommended for patients who have a persistent elevation of diastolic blood pressure over 90 millimeters of mercury in readings taken on three different occasions.

Two factors which are associated with a tendency to raise the blood pressure are excessive salt intake and obesity. Treatment for mild to moderate hypertension begins with diet. Indeed, the diet is important in any hypertensive patient, even those on medication. Reduction of salt or sodium intake and maintenance of ideal body weight are dietary goals of all individuals with hypertension.

If there is a tendency to hypertension, it may be made worse by severe stressful conditions or by excessive loss of sleep. In some patients with hypertension, it may be advisable to suggest a change in life style.

If sodium restriction and weight reduction do not reduce the blood pressure below 90 to 95 millimeters of mercury, then a drug should be taken. Drug treatment of hypertension usually begins with the use of a diuretic, most often from the thiazide family. These drugs have been used for a number of years and are relatively safe, although an excessive loss of potassium occurs in some patients. Some drugs are long-acting and need to be taken only once a day. If diet plus the thiazide does not satisfactorily reduce the blood pressure, a variety of other agents may be added such as olphamethyldopa or propanalol. Virtually all drugs have side effects and therefore close medical supervision is mandatory. Medical monitoring of the blood pressure also is required to make certain that the regimen being prescribed is effective. New drugs are available—a few only on an experimental basis—which have considerable promise.

One of the greatest problems in treating hypertension is to get the patient to take the medication properly. It is important to realize that a drug is effective only as long as it is taken. That is, if the medication is not taken on a regular schedule, the blood pressure will rise again.

In conclusion, we believe that hypertension is one of the most important risk factors in cardiovascular disease. If more than one risk factor is present, the seriousness of hypertension is greater. Therefore, for patients with high blood pressure, it is very important to control this problem, but it is also desirable to eliminate cigarette smoking and make sure that the serum cholesterol level is not elevated. It is of the utmost importance to have the blood pressure checked annually. We agree with the American Heart Association which has promoted mass blood pressure screening and has encouraged public participation through its appeal to "perform a death-defying act."

15

ARTIFICIAL PACEMAKERS, CARDIAC SUPPORT AND REPLACEMENT

L_{ET} us review the electrical conduction system of the heart which has been discussed at length in Chapter 14. Electrical impulses originate in the sinoatrial (SA) node of the right atrium, pass through the myocardial fibers of the right and left atria and activate the AV node (Figure 113). From the AV node, electrical activity travels through the bundle of His in the muscular septum between the ventricles. The bundle divides into right and left bundle branches which fan out over the left and right ventricles. As the electrical impulses pass through the atria, they induce contraction of these chambers. When they reach the ventricular muscle fibers, they cause contraction of the ventricles. Interference with the conduction system at one or more sites can produce first-degree, second-degree, or third-degree heart block as described in Chapter 4.

In order to understand why and when artificial pacemakers are recommended, the various types of heart block must be discussed. First-degree AV block is a delay in the transmission of an electrical impulse from the atrium to the ventricle. All impulses are transmitted so there is little or no

201

decrease in the heart rate or change in its regularity. First-degree AV block may be caused by fibrosis of the conduction system or by drugs; it is rarely an indication for the insertion of a pacemaker.

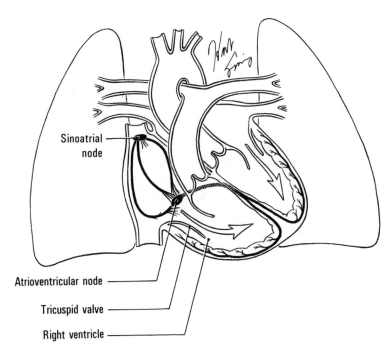

Figure 113. The electrical conduction system of the normal heart

Second-degree AV block is of two types. In Type I, there is a progressive delay in the electrical transmission until an impulse is blocked from entering the ventricle. Thus the atria may beat three times while the ventricle beats only twice. This form of heart block is usually reversible and occurs after myocardial infarction or in response to an excessive amount of digitalis. Type II second-degree AV heart block has a different pattern. In this condition the impulse may be transmitted without delay one time and not at all the next. Type II AV block is often unstable and may suddenly progress to third-degree block; it is an indication for pacemaker insertion.

Third-degree AV block (complete AV dissociation or complete heart block), except when it is congenital, is a serious condition. The electrical activity that triggers contraction begins in the ventricles themselves and thus is slow and unstable. When the block occurs suddenly, it will often cause a sudden loss of consciousness (Stokes-Adams attack). The life expectancy of a patient with acquired complete heart block is significantly decreased. Although pacemakers may increase longevity, life expectancy is also determined by the underlying condition which led to the heart block. When it occurs as a consequence of an acute myocardial infarction, the prognosis is worse than when it is secondary to fibrosis. In either case, however, pacemaker insertion improves the quality of life and allows maintenance of an adequate circulation to the vital organs.

The great majority of pacemakers now used are implanted in the patient and are of the transvenous type, which can be inserted without opening the chest (Figure 114). The electrodes of the transvenous intracardiac pacemaker

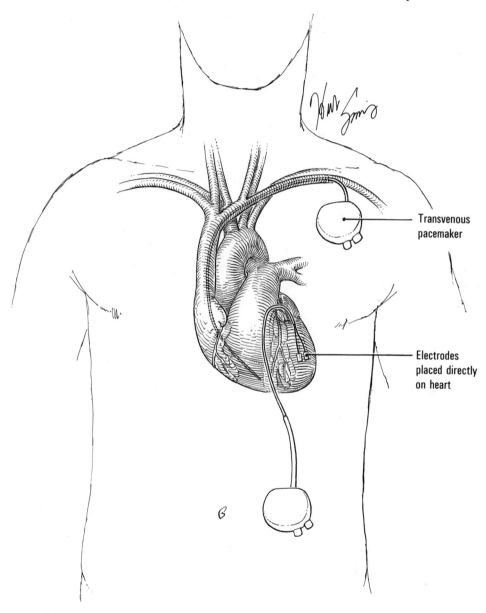

Transvenous pacemaker

Electrodes placed directly on heart

Figure 114. Two commonly used artificial pacemakers

are positioned in the right ventricle by passing them into a peripheral vein, usually the external jugular or cephalic. From the vein they are passed through the superior vena cava, into the right atrium and finally, to the apex of the right ventricle. The batteries are placed under the skin below the clavicle, or collar bone. Thus, a very simple procedure, not requiring opening the chest, is used to put the transvenous pacemaker in place. An alternate method of pacemaker insertion requires opening of the chest to place the electrodes directly on the heart muscle, near the apex of the left ventricle. In addition to the incision in the chest wall, a second incision is made either in the abdomen or armpit. A tunnel is made beneath the skin and underlying fat in order to pass the electrode from the left ventricle to the battery which is placed at the site of the second incision.

There are two basic types of pacemakers: asynchronous and synchronous, or demand. The asynchronous pacemaker discharges at fixed intervals to stimulate the heart at a fixed rate. Even if the intrinsic rate of the heart exceeds the rate of the pacemaker, the pacemaker will continue to discharge. The demand or synchronous pacemaker fires only when the heart rate falls below a predetermined rate, usually sixty-eight to seventy-two beats per minute and, for this reason, is the most widely used.

In an emergency situation where immediate pacing is required, a method for temporary pacing is available. Most often a pacing or electrode catheter is inserted through a peripheral vein and guided into the right ventricle. It then is attached to an external power source. Pacing may also be accomplished by placing two electrodes on the chest wall over the heart and applying a much higher voltage. This method is less reliable and often very unpleasant for the patient.

An average pacemaker is about one-inch thick, just under three inches in diameter and weighs approximately five ounces. Power sources used in most pacemakers usually require replacement every two to three years, although new developments in power sources and patient surveillance may prolong the life of the generator. Recently, a nuclear-powered generator has been developed as an effort to offer a long-term energy supply.

Occasional complications that occur with a pacemaker usually can be dealt with by the patient's physician. Some of these include infection of the wound, displacement of the electrodes or a random failure of a part of this complicated mechanical device. The risk of these complications may be minimized by a regular schedule of visits to the doctor or pacemaker clinic.

Some patients become overly aware of the presence of the pacemaker inside their chest and liken it to a time bomb. When this happens, the best approach is for the patient to discuss the situation with his physician, obtain reassurance and begin a regulated program of physical activity. This program should be gradually increased to a point where the patient is able to carry out a normal routine of activity. There should be no problem in driving a car and traveling as one pleases. Concern about the possibility that

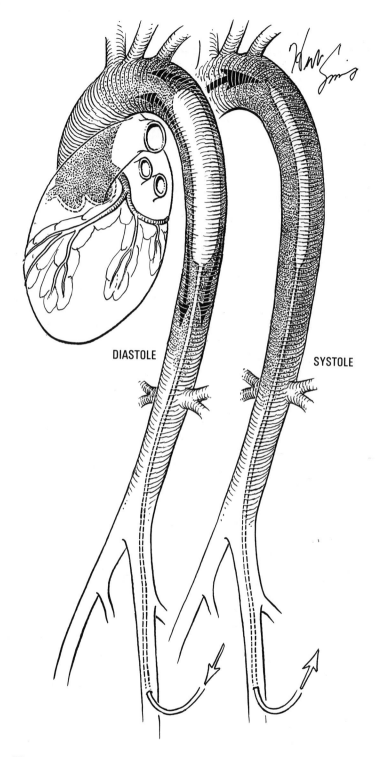

DIASTOLE

SYSTOLE

Figure 115. The use of an intra-aortic balloon to assist the heart in pumping blood throughout the body

electrical equipment can cause pacemaker dysfunction has probably been exaggerated. Most problems are related to industrial exposure. Each individual should discuss his particular activities with his physician. The use of pacemakers has been one of the most significant advances in the cardiovascular field in the past fifteen years.

Circulatory Assist Devices and the Artificial Heart

The need for devising a mechanism for assisting the failing heart was recognized long ago. More than three-quarters of patients who have heart attacks and develop shock or hypotension do not survive. Research and development of devices and techniques for assisting the failing left ventricle has received a high priority by the government and the National Heart, Lung and Blood Institute over the past decade. Since the essence of the function of the heart muscle is to pump the blood to the tissues of the body, it was logical to think in terms of constructing an artificial heart in the form of a pump. In the late 1950s, several articles published in medical journals described the development of artificial devices aimed at replacing the function of the heart.

Further attempts at developing ventricular-assist devices resulted in the production of basic designs which used electrical, hydraulic or skeletal muscle as a source of power. The use of such devices in animals or human beings introduces a number of physiological and biochemical problems. These include the destruction of blood cells, clotting of the blood, deposition of materials from the blood within the device, wear and tear of the machine, interference with normal regulatory feedback mechanisms and the immunological response of the host to the foreign material. Such a perplexing array of problems has required a broad-based attack by teams of investigators representing a variety of medical, engineering, biological and other scientific disciplines.

There are four basic principles for assisting the failing heart. One is external cardiac massage. Several techniques have been developed to apply cardiac massage directly to the surface of the heart. However, in contrast to cardiopulmonary resuscitation, which is a non-invasive technique, direct cardiac massage requires opening the chest, which is a major disadvantage to the patient suffering from a heart attack and in shock. The basic principle is to apply a cup with a diaphragm around the heart and administer alternate positive and negative pressure to assist in the emptying and filling of the left ventricle. This method has a number of disadvantages and is therefore not generally employed.

A second procedure is referred to as counterpulsation and it is most often accomplished with an intra-aortic balloon, which is alternately inflated and deflated (Figure 115). Deflation during systole decreases resistance against which the heart has to pump and increases the capacity of the aorta to hold

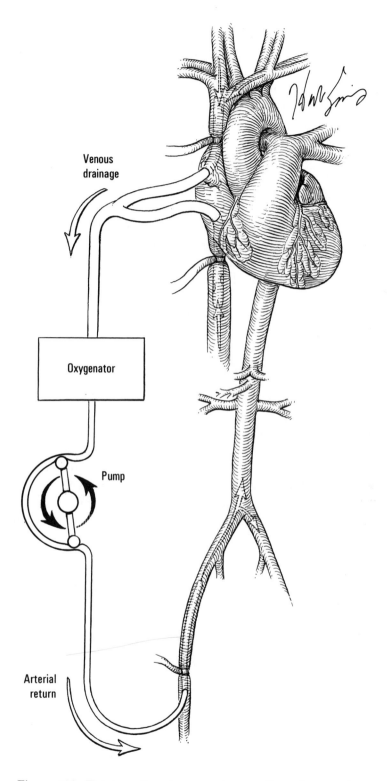

Figure 116. Total cardiopulmonary bypass (heart-lung machine) during open-heart surgery

blood. During diastole, the balloon is inflated to displace the blood pumped by the heart. The resultant higher diastolic pressure increases blood flow to the brain, coronary arteries and kidneys. Such a device increases oxygen consumption by the heart and reduces its work load. This method is being used with some success in a number of centers throughtout the country, including our Cardiovascular Center at The Methodist Hospital in Houston. Its advantages lie in its relatively simple, low-risk application, since it can be applied using a local anesthetic. Its most common application has been in patients with severe heart failure and shock following an acute heart attack that does not respond to standard medical treatment.

The third method of providing temporary cardiac assistance is with the use of the heart-lung machine. Total cardiopulmonary bypass, using the heart-lung machine, has revolutionized open-heart surgery (Figure 116). Application of total or partial cardiopulmonary bypass with the heart-lung machine is limited to about five or six hours because of damage to the red blood cells and the plasma proteins. The development of a device called the membrane oxygenator has decreased the turbulence produced at the interface at which the gas exchange occurs. During total cardiopulmonary bypass, the action of pumping blood by the heart is completely replaced by the heart-lung machine.

As a patient is taken off total cardiopulmonary bypass, the tourniquets around the superior and inferior venae cavae are released and blood flow to the right side of the heart resumes. Blood flow to the left ventricle increases and, for a time, the heart and lungs work in parallel with the pump oxygenator. The amount of blood going through the machine is gradually decreased until the heart and lungs completely take over their functions of pumping and oxygenating blood. If the left ventricle cannot resume its work load, heart failure ensues and the ventricular cavity is not emptied completely. Pressure in the left ventricle during diastole then increases, which results in a decreased filling from the left atrium (Figure 117). This in turn increases pressure back to the lungs and causes congestion there. A vicious cycle ensues; the oxygen supply to the tissues is decreased and unless reversed, low blood pressure, low cardiac output, tissue hypoxia and death will result.

Total cardiopulmonary bypass as a means of temporary cardiac assist has a number of disadvantages, including the need for a major operation and general anesthetic. The five or six hours limit to the time it can be used may not be sufficient time for the heart to recover. Therefore, it is usually applied only in cases that necessitate an operation for correction of a cause of heart failure, such as valvular disease. Its success as a temporary support of the circulation following completion of the surgical procedure is dependent upon the ability of the left ventricle to recover adequate function within a matter of four to six hours.

When the damaged left ventricle is unable to recover after four to six hours, there are other methods of circulatory support that can be used. Most

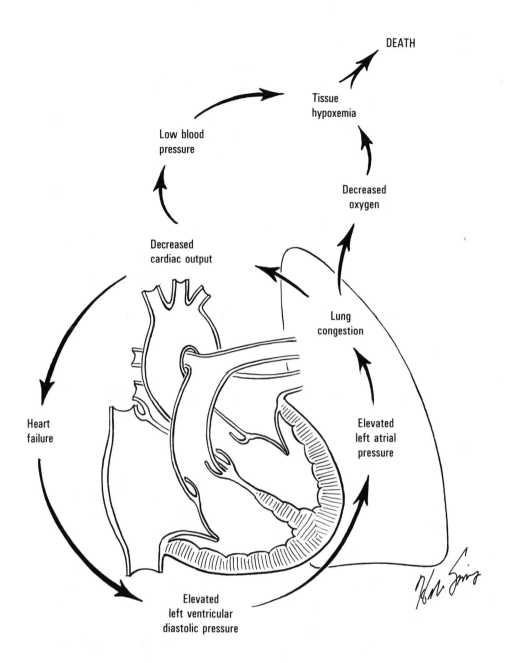

DEATH

Tissue
hypoxemia

Low blood
pressure

Decreased
oxygen

Decreased
cardiac output

Lung
congestion

Heart
failure

Elevated
left atrial
pressure

Elevated
left ventricular
diastolic pressure

Figure 117. The "vicious cycle" of heart failure

of them are based upon the principle of removing blood from the left atrium or left ventricle by a tube and then using an artificial pump to return the blood to the arterial system by a tube that is connected to a major artery (Figure 118). This assist device is called a left ventricular bypass pump.

Following considerable experimental work, the first left ventricular bypass pump was implanted in a patient at the Cardiovascular Center of The Methodist Hospital in 1963; this device pumped the blood from the left atrium into the descending thoracic aorta. Although this patient subsequently died from brain damage that had previously occurred, there was evidence that the bypass pump functioned in assisting the left ventricle. Further experimental work led to the development of a left ventricular bypass pump that was successfully used for the first time on August 8, 1966. The patient, a thirty-seven-year-old woman with severe heart failure resulting from rheumatic aortic and mitral valve disease, required surgical replacement of both valves. Following completion of the operation using artificial valves to replace the damaged ones, the left ventricle was unable to resume adequate function without the support of the heart-lung machine. The left ventricular bypass pump was then attached by connecting tubes to the left atrium and the right axillary artery (Figure 118). With this method of supporting the left ventricle it was then possible to take the patient off the heart-lung machine. After ten days of support by the left ventricular bypass pump, the left ventricle recovered enough to allow removal of the assist

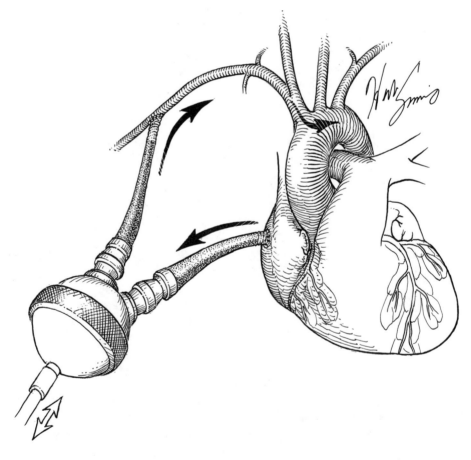

Figure 118. The DeBakey left ventricular bypass pump used to assist the failing heart to pump blood throughout the body

device. The patient recovered completely and resumed normal life for about six years, until she was tragically killed in an automobile accident.

The left ventricular bypass pump takes oxygenated blood from the left atrium, and pumps it back into the arterial circulation by a connection to the ascending aorta or to a major peripheral artery such as the femoral or axillary artery. Left atrial pressure, pressure in the left ventricle and pulmonary congestion are reduced. Blood may be pumped during diastole, when the

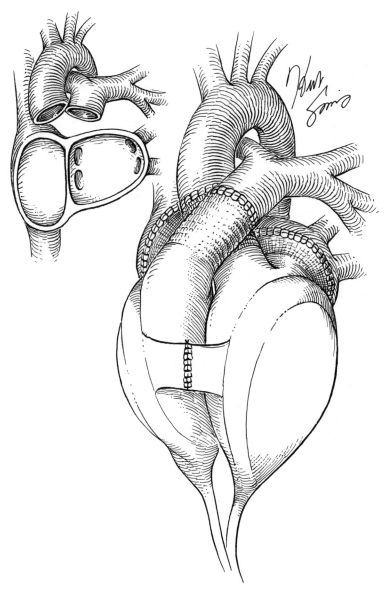

Figure 119. The total cardiac prosthesis (artificial heart) consists of two bypass pumps which replace the functions of the two ventricles of the natural heart.

aortic valve is closed, to increase perfusion of the coronary arteries and aid in the recovery of the damaged myocardium. In contrast to the heart-lung machine, the design of the left ventricular bypass pump allows two to three liters of blood per minute to be pumped for a prolonged period of time with little damage to the blood and its elements.

The bypass pump consists of an outer rigid plastic material somewhat hemispherical in shape. Two inner chambers are separated by a flexible plastic diaphragm. One of these chambers is for blood and the other is for gas. The blood chamber has two openings with ball valves which serve as the entrance and the exit for the tubes from the left atrium and to the artery. When pressurized carbon dioxide gas is pulsed into the gas chamber, the flexible diaphragm collapses the blood chamber, forcing blood into the tubing connected to the artery. When the pressure in the gas chamber is released, blood is allowed to fill the blood chamber from the heart. The regular, continuous repetition of this process pumps blood in a manner much like the natural left ventricle. The pump and tubing is lined with Dacron velour, a material used for artificial arteries. This allows firm adherence of a fibrinous material which is deposited on the velour surfaces from the blood. The resulting surface is quite compatible with the blood and greatly reduces damage to its various elements. Unfortunately, after several weeks there is a tendency for the surface to progressively thicken, which ultimately interferes with blood flow through the chamber and tubings. But for several weeks it may function satisfactorily, and this is a sufficient period of time to permit the heart to recover if it possibly can.

The major disadvantage of this method of cardiac assistance lies in the fact that its application requires a major operation, and it is therefore limited to patients whose cardiac disease requires surgery.

Total replacement of the heart with an artificial pumping device is an ultimate goal for helping the patient with irreversible heart failure (Figure 119). Replacing the two pumping chambers of the heart requires the solution of enormous biological problems as well as advances in fabrication, materials, and power supply. Development of a successful artificial heart will require patient, long-term approaches and many years of research and development.

Transplantation

Transplantation of the human heart has probably evoked as much controversy as any subject in the history of cardiovascular disease. Pioneering work on heart transplantation was done in animals in the early part of the twentieth century by Dr. Alexis Carrell and Dr. Charles C. Guthrie, and more recently by Dr. Norman Shumway at Stanford University. Dr. Christian Barnard performed the first successful human heart transplant on December 3, 1967, in Capetown, South Africa, at the Groote Schuur Hospital. After an initial flourish of activity in many centers, the enthusiasm for this operation declined, except for Dr. Shumway's group at Stanford. As had previously occurred with kidney transplants, as Dr. Shumway's group gained more experience with heart transplantation, the survival rate improved. It is possible that in some cases, the individual recipient develops a type of blocking antibody which retards rejection of the transplanted heart by antibodies produced in the recipient's body.

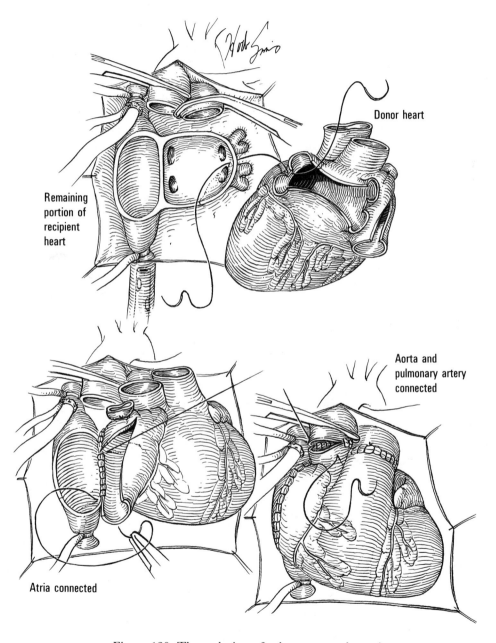

Figure 120. The technique for heart transplantation

Heart transplantation is a last resort for a patient with intractable heart failure. The donor and the recipient are tested for compatibility of their tissues by checking their blood types and lymphocytes. There must be complete compatibility with respect to blood types. The tissue compatibility, obtained by matching their lymphocytes, is assigned a value on a graded scale. The majority of recipients of heart transplantations have used donors who fall approximately in the middle of the tissue compatability scale. The donor is usually an individual who has irreversible brain damage from a accident or some other cause. Many ethical considerations are involved. The donor must be pronounced dead. A set of criteria for the determination of death has been proposed and widely discussed. If the transplantation is to be successful, the donor's heart must be kept viable. The recipient is attached to the heart-lung machine and placed on total cardiopulmonary bypass. The recipient's heart is then removed, leaving intact the posterior parts of the atria and the openings of the aorta and pulmonary artery (Figure 120). At the same time, the heart of the donor is removed, placed in a cold salt solution and taken to the recipient. The atria of the donor are trimmed to fit the remaining portion of the atria of the recipient. The donor heart is then placed in the pericardial cavity of the recipient. The edges of the left atrial wall of the donor are sewn to the edges of the remaining left atrial wall of the receipient; a similar attachment is made for the right atrium. The open end of the pulmonary artery of the donor heart is then attached by suture to the open end of the pulmonary artery of the recipient. The aorta of the donor heart is similarly connected to the aorta of the recipient. All nervous connections of the heart, both parasympathetic and sympathetic, are severed during the operation. The heart is restarted by defibrillation and electrical activity is resumed by the donor heart's intrinsic pacemaker and electrical conduction system. Since the sinoatrial node of the recipient is preserved and that of the donor is intact, the electrocardiogram may show atrial electrical activity from both recipient and donor hearts.

Our experience with heart transplants is limited to twelve patients, of which ten died of rejection or related complications in less than one year. Of the two remaining patients, one survived for about four years and the other about six years, before dying of chronic rejection. Until their deaths, both patients were active and led reasonably normal lives.

On the basis of this experience and for a number of other reasons, we at the Cardiovascular Center of The Methodist Hospital, like most surgeons, discontinued performing the procedure. Immunological rejection of the transplanted heart by the recipient remains a major problem, both as an immediate and as a later cause of death. The cost of the operation in terms of specialized personnel, facilities, equipment and immediate and post-operative care is prohibitive for most centers. The availability of donors is a major problem, since this is dependent upon a rather special type of accident in which the heart is not damaged, but where death occurs from brain damage.

During the period when we were performing heart transplants we had many patients who died waiting for such a tragic accident to occur in order to obtain a donor. For this reason, even if the immunological rejection problem were solved, which does not seem likely in the foreseeable future, the operation would have only limited application. Currently, only a few heart centers, the most notable being the one at Stanford University, continue to perform the operation.

16

DISEASES

OF

THE VEINS

A common miscomprehension by patients is that atherosclerosis affects both the arterial and the venous systems. This is not correct. Except in rare instances, atherosclerosis or arteriosclerosis as discussed in this book is limited to the arterial system. A patient may have severe atherosclerosis with normal veins, venous disease with normal arteries or disease of both the arterial and the venous systems. Diseases which affect the veins, the subject of this chapter, are nonatherosclerotic unless part of the venous system is subjected to arterial pressure.

While blood flow in the arterial system is propelled by the heart and takes place under high pressure, the pressure in the venous system is ordinarily quite low. Blood is returned to the heart through the low-pressure venous system by external compression from muscular movements, which propel the flow from the peripheries through unidirectional valves. Under pathological conditions, the level of venous pressure may be greatly increased. For example, in the patient with pulmonary hypertension, the pulmonary veins are subjected to a high pressure and develop severe atherosclerotic changes. Thus, it is probable that it is the relative low pressure that protects the venous system from the development of atherosclerosis.

Surgical techniques that have been successful in the treatment of arterial disease have failed when used on the venous system. Methods for replacing the diseased valves of veins have not met with success. Nor has it been possible to use grafts in the venous system with much success, since they become occluded from thrombosis or from the deposition of fibrous connective tissue.

The most common problem affecting the venous system is varicose veins. The varicosities occur mainly in the network of saphenous veins in the legs. They are caused by incompetence of the valves, which permits backflow or leakage, or by occlusion in the deep system of veins within the legs. Treatment of this condition is less complicated if the disease is located primarily within the saphenous system itself and the deep veins are uninvolved. Conservative treatment includes avoiding prolonged standing or crossing of the legs. Fitted elastic support stockings may be very useful. Surgical treatment of this disease is limited to the superficial saphenous system. It consists of tying off or stripping away the diseased portion of vein or of injecting a sclerosing solution to obliterate its lumen. There is sufficient collateral circulation so that the ligated, excised or sclerosed segment of the vein will not lead to venous congestion in the extremity. If the venous disease progresses to the point that ulceration of the skin develops, skin grafting may be required.

A much more serious situation occurs when there is thrombosis of the deep veins of the leg. Rudolf Virchow originally presented an hypothesis of venous thromboembolism over 125 years ago. He thought that venous thrombosis resulted from damage to the wall of the vein, due to changes in the blood and sluggishness of circulation, which promoted coagulation.

An embolus is a portion of a thrombus, or clot, that breaks off and is carried to a distant part of the circulatory system where it lodges in another blood vessel. An embolus from the veins of the lower extremities usually lodges in the lungs and is referred to as a pulmonary embolus. Even today, the precise causes of venous thrombosis and of pulmonary embolism have not been defined. Patients immobilized for periods of time, those who have stasis of blood due to varicosities, congestive heart failure or pregnancy, those having trauma to the extremities, or those with an increased number of red blood cells and various types of malignancies, all show an enhanced tendency to develop thrombosis of the deep veins of the legs. An inflammatory phase associated with thrombosis is referred to as phlebitis or thrombophlebitis or phlebothrombosis. The thrombosis and inflammation may be primarily superficial, deep or both. The clinical manifestations may be mild to severe and pulmonary embolism can be a dangerous complication. On rare occasions there may be a massive reaction in the leg, progressing to severe edema and inflammation. This occurs with thrombosis of the iliofemoral vein because of its anatomic location. The patient in such cases is acutely ill and death may ensue or the extremity may be lost. Long-term complications include venous insufficiency of the extremity and recurrent bouts of thrombophlebitis.

Thrombophlebitis of either the superficial or deep venous system should be treated with bed rest, elevation and wrapping of the legs, and anticoagulation with the drug heparin. In some instances, venous thrombectomy, that is, the direct surgical removal of the venous thrombosis, may be lifesaving. Such surgical treatment should be performed as soon as possible for iliofemoral thrombosis.

The first venous thrombectomy was reported by M. Demons of Bordeaux, France in 1881. The techniques currently employed are similar to those used for *embolectomy* of an artery. For thrombosis of the iliofemoral veins, the common femoral vein is exposed by an incision in the groin. In many patients, this exposure will allow complete removal of all of the thrombotic material. In other patients, it may be necessary to expose the inferior vena cava through an abdominal incision. Treatment with heparin is continued after the operation.

The treatment of pulmonary emboli requires special consideration aimed at preventing recurrence. Fortunately, most of these emboli are small. Treatment of the acute attack consists of bed rest, elevation and wrapping of the legs, and anticoagulation. Anticoagulant treatment is continued after the acute period. If the patient has a further pulmonary embolus while on anticoagulants, or if for some reason these drugs cannot be used, it may then become necessary to interrupt the venous system at the level of the inferior vena cava to prevent a recurrence of embolization. The thrombosis usually extends up into the inferior vena cava so that ligation at a level below the vena cava is not satisfactory.

In the patient with a massive acute pulmonary embolism, it may be necessary to perform an embolectomy as an emergency, lifesaving measure. This procedure was originally suggested in 1908 by Friedrich Trendelenburg. The first successful surgery to treat an acute massive pulmonary embolism by an embolectomy using a temporary cardiopulmonary bypass was performed at the Cardiovascular Center of The Methodist Hospital in 1961. This approach allows enough time to permit clearing of the emboli from the pulmonary artery and subsequently has been used successfully on a number of patients.

Further significant advances in surgery of the venous system will demand procedures that allow grafting or the replacement of damaged valves within the vein.

17

PREVENTIVE
MAINTENANCE

APPROXIMATELY fifteen million people in the United States suffer from some form of cardiovascular disease, and one million of them die each year. About 700,000 of these deaths are from myocardial infarctions, or heart attacks. Over one-half of the deaths in America, approximately 54 percent, are from cardiovascular disease, now the leading cause of death and disability in our society. Thus, practically every American is touched, directly or indirectly, by this number-one public health problem. It is likely that one out of two readers of this book will die of some form of heart disease.

There is some hope from preliminary data which suggests that the death rate from coronary artery disease in the United States has peaked and may have actually begun to decline over the past ten years. Unfortunately, we do not know enough to identify which changes occurred in the American population to account for this apparent decline.

There is no way to be immunized against cardiovascular disease. However, there are well-recognized risk factors which may make it more likely that an individual will have a heart attack or stroke at an early age

(Figure 121). It should be emphasized that at this time there is no direct scientific proof that correction of these risk factors will decrease the risk of cardiovascular death. In any case, it seems wise to take steps to eliminate them if they are present.

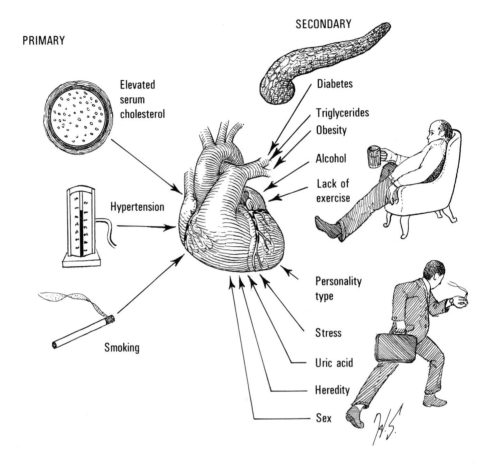

Figure 121. The risk factors in arteriosclerosis

Most cardiovascular catastrophes are caused by atherosclerosis. Perhaps in as many as 75 percent of the people who die or who are disabled from this disease and its complications, one or more of three primary risk factors are present. These are 1) elevations of serum or blood cholesterol; 2) elevation of blood pressure, or hypertension; and 3) cigarette smoking.

Primary Risk Factors

Elevated Serum Cholesterol (and Serum Triglycerides). Cholesterol and triglyceride are blood fats or lipids. When present in the blood in excessive concentrations, the patient is said to have *hyperlipidemia*. The relationship between elevated blood cholesterol and atherosclerosis follows logically from the detailed discussion in Chapter 8. The cholesterol that accumulates within the arterial wall and contributes to the formation of an atheromatous plaque, is derived from the plasma where it is carried by the lipoproteins. In the mid-nineteenth century, Rudolf Virchow (1821–1902), a German pathologist, observed cheesy, fatlike material built up along the interior walls of atherosclerotic blood vessels when viewed under a microscope. Virchow and his colleagues eventually identified cholesterol as a major lipid constituent in these lesions. Other scientists subsequently have obtained evidence to support the conclusion that the blood is the major source of the cholesterol that accumulates within the wall of the arteries. Individuals with high levels of cholesterol in the blood are at greater risk for developing premature heart attacks and other atherosclerotic complications than are individuals with low or normal levels. A major population study concerning the risk associated with a high serum cholesterol was carried out in Framingham, Massachusetts. It may be concluded that for a man between the ages of thirty and fifty, an elevation of serum cholesterol over 260 milligrams percent increases the risk of developing coronary artery disease in the next five years by three and one-half times or more as compared to the risk with a cholesterol level less than 200 milligrams percent.

It has long been thought that there probably is a connection between diet, serum cholesterol and coronary heart disease. For example, there was a marked decrease in coronary heart disease death rates in parts of Scandinavia, Belgium, the Netherlands and Leningrad during periods of food shortage in World War II. Wartime shortages of meat and dairy products decreased the consumption of cholesterol and unsaturated fat.

For a number of years, it was thought by many physicians that serum cholesterol could not be lowered by diet. This view arose from the discovery that animals have a negative feedback system to regulate cholesterol synthesis in the liver. The more cholesterol present in the diet, the less cholesterol the liver makes. Conversely, the more the dietary cholesterol is restricted, the more cholesterol the liver produces. The cholesterol that circulates in the blood thus has two origins. Some is derived from the diet while the rest is synthesized in the body, primarily in the liver and intestine. However, there is now indisputable evidence that serum cholesterol can be lowered at least 10 to 15 percent by making relatively simple modifications in the diet.

While obesity is a risk factor that tends to aggravate other risk factors, such as high blood pressure and high blood triglycerides, obesity per se does not have a major effect on the concentration of serum cholesterol. There are three dietary factors which are very important in regulating the cholesterol level in the blood. They are the amounts of polyunsaturated fat, saturated fat and cholesterol in the diet. We will refer to the dietary ratio of polyunsaturated to saturated fat as the P/S ratio. Saturated fats tend to be solid at room temperature, while the more unsaturated fats tend to be liquid. Dairy products, most meats and particularly organ meats, are very rich in saturated fat and/or cholesterol. Certain meats, such as fish, poultry and veal, are not as rich in saturated fats as are beef and pork. The only types of fish that are excluded for patients on a cholesterol-restricted diet are shrimp and crayfish. Most shellfish were formerly restricted, but more recent analysis of lipid composition by the U.S. Department of Agriculture has led to a revision of dietary recommendations.

Whereas the average American diet has a P/S ratio of about 0.3, in order to obtain lower cholesterol, the ratio should be 1.0 or greater. To accomplish this, it is necessary to use vegetable oils rather than lard or butter for cooking. The vegetable oil richest in polyunsaturated fat is safflower oil, followed by corn and sunflower seed oils, soybean and cottonseed oils, and then peanut and olive oils. Margarine is much richer in polyunsaturated fat than is butter. In general, the softer the margarine the higher the P/S ratio. Skim milk and low fat milk also contain less saturated fat than whole milk and cream. One of the richest sources of cholesterol in the American diet is egg yolk. The average daily American intake of cholesterol is 600 to 800 milligrams. The average egg yolk contains 250 to 300 milligrams and thus represents a significant contribution to the daily cholesterol intake.

We recommend that all our patients have the serum cholesterol checked to determine whether or not it is high. This can be done through a simple blood test; the triglycerides should be checked at the same time. The tests should be done after the patient has fasted for twelve hours, has been on a regular diet prior to the fast, is neither losing nor gaining weight, is not acutely ill, and is not taking medication that will either raise or lower the blood fats. One of the worst times to measure cholesterol or triglycerides is immediately after a heart attack. It is desirable to wait at least three weeks after a heart attack before checking the blood fats, cholesterol or triglycerides.

At the present time we do not know what constitutes a safe level of cholesterol. We would recommend that if the cholesterol is over 250 milligrams percent, a vigorous dietary program aimed at reducing this elevation should be instituted. For intermediate levels of 200 to 250 milligrams percent, or for the interested patient who wishes to reduce the concentration, we recommend a moderate degree of restriction of dietary cholesterol and saturated fat. It is interesting to note that in countries where the serum cholesterol is less than 150 milligrams percent, atherosclerosis is practically nonexistent.

For a prudent diet, we recommend that the overall cholesterol intake be limited to not more than 300 milligrams per day. This allows the weekly consumption of two to three eggs, including those used in cooking. A similar diet has been recommended by the American Heart Association. We advise our patients to read the labels on foods carefully. The Voluntary Labeling Act of 1974 permits the manufacturer to give the consumer a great deal of useful information about the composition of food. The ratio of polyunsaturated fat to saturated fat as well as the cholesterol content should be checked. For margarines, the manufacturer is required by law to list the ingredients in the order of their quantities. Therefore, the first ingredient listed on the margarine label should be a natural vegetable oil, such as corn oil. On many margarines the first ingredient is a partially hydrogenated or partially saturated vegetable oil. Such margarines are less effective in contributing to an increase in the polyunsaturated fat content of the diet.

It should be emphasized that no one food alone is the villain causing heart disease or provides the key to preventing heart attack. Claims that a particular food will protect you against heart disease are misleading.

It is possible to lower serum cholesterol in patients with elevated levels through the use of drugs such as cholestryamine, nicotinic acid and clofibrate. The drug acts in addition to the effect of the diet. However, as with diet, it is not known whether lowering cholesterol with medication will protect against cardiovascular disease. It is hoped that this question will be resolved by the Coronary Primary Prevention Trial of the Lipid Research Clinics Program of the National Heart, Lung and Blood Institute.

We have listed the serum triglycerides as a secondary risk factor, but now will discuss it in conjunction with cholesterol since both are blood *lipids,* or fats. The evidence linking elevated triglycerides to coronary heart disease is not as strong as it is for serum cholesterol. The triglycerides may be solid, such as lard, or even liquid, like corn oil or safflower oil. The more unsaturated the fatty acids of the triglyceride, the greater is the tendency to be a liquid. There are many studies that report an increased incidence of coronary heart disease in patients with elevated levels of serum triglycerides. As with cholesterol, the triglycerides in the bloodstream may be derived either from the diet or from synthesis by the body. An elevation of serum triglycerides is extremely common in the American population. Two of the major contributors to this problem are obesity and excessive consumption of alcohol. In some patients, a high carbohydrate intake, particularly of sugar, may contribute to the hypertriglyceridemia. Insulin deficiency also raises the consumption to two ounces of spirits per day, and to limit the intake of sweets an elevation of triglycerides to reduce to ideal body weight, to restrict alcohol and sugar. We do not recommend severe restrictions of carbohydrate. Most cases of elevated serum triglycerides can be normalized by a simple change in the diet. It may be necessary to use a drug in addition to the diet for some patients.

It has been found that some individuals have an inherited tendency to high levels of serum cholesterol, triglycerides or both. Several different inherited disorders have been identified. Three of the most common varieties are familial hypercholesterolemia (or Type II hyperlipidemia), familial hypertriglyceridemia (Type IV hyperlipidemia), and familial combined hyperlipidemia, in which both cholesterol and triglycerides are elevated (usually Type IIB hyperlipidemia). In such individuals there is an increased tendency to oversynthesize the lipid or its carrier, lipoprotein, or an inability to clear it from the blood at a normal rate or a combination of both problems. In one study carried out in Seattle, Washington, about one out of three survivors of myocardial infarctions had some form of familial hyperlipidemia. Most patients with elevated serum cholesterols do not, however, have familial hypercholesterolemia—perhaps only one out of ten. Because the problem may be inherited, we recommend that children of parents with elevated serum lipids be screened to determine whether or not they are affected.

In many of the patients with inherited forms of hyperlipidemia, diet alone may be insufficient to control the problem. There are relatively safe, effective medications available, and they are used in conjunction with a diet. Before taking a medication for hyperlipidemia, the specific type of blood disorder should be diagnosed, secondary causes such as hypothyroidism must be excluded, and a conscientious effort should be made to control the problem by treatment with diet.

Hypertension. (See Chapter 14.) One of the most common of the primary risk factors for cardiovascular disease—and probably the most neglected—is hypertension. It is the single most important risk factor for stroke or a cerebrovascular accident.

For patients with a tendency toward hypertension, salt in the diet can be particularly troublesome. Doctor Walter Kempner popularized the use of the rice diet for hypertension a number of years ago. The effectiveness of this diet is related to its low salt content.   •

Cigarette Smoking. Smoking was not a major problem in the United States prior to World War II. Two technical advances led to the widespread use of cigarettes. One was the development of an effective and economical way of mass producing cigarettes; the second was the improvement of the cigarette so as to make it less acidic and more appealing.

The dangers of smoking now are pointed out on each package of cigarettes as a result of the Surgeon General's report on smoking issued in 1964. Most Americans are aware of the relationship of smoking to lung cancer and other respiratory diseases. It is not as well know that smoking is one of the three primary risk factors for cardiovascular disease. Doctor Alton Ochsner, chairman of the Department of Surgery at Tulane University Medical School, once said, "Smoking may have at least one virtue. By smoking heavily a man may have a heart attack, then he would not live long enough to develop cancer." Unfortunately, the nonsmoker is subjected to nicotine by exposure to the smoker. The level of nicotine in the blood of the nonsmoker may approximate 5 percent of that in the smoker.

The precise way in which smoking leads to cardiovascular death is not known. Nicotine is released into the blood and may have a toxic effect on the muscle cells of the heart or arterioles. Smoking also increases the carbon monoxide content of the blood, which displaces oxygen from hemoglobin and can reduce the oxygen supply to vulnerable, peripheral tissues, including the blood vessels. In the case of preexisting arteriosclerosis, cigarette smoking may hasten the development of a coronary occlusion or the occlusion of blood vessels in other areas. It has long been a common clinical observation that cigarette smoking aggravates a form of peripheral arteriosclerosis referred to as Buerger's disease. Many who have stopped smoking have reported an improvement in the symptoms of this disease. A five-year study conducted at the Mayo Clinic demonstrated the benefit of quitting cigarette smoking in patients with peripheral arterial occlusive disease.

Since the Surgeon General's pronouncement against smoking, there has been a drastic reduction in cigarette smoking by physicians and a significant decrease in middle-aged men. Unfortunately, the decrease by adults has been offset by an increase in young people and women. This situation seems to reflect a deficiency in our educational systems. An effective program is needed to educate the public, particularly school children, about the hazards of taking up the habit. We need to learn which factors influence a person to smoke and which keep people from beginning in the first place. We already know that if one or both parents smoke, a youngster is much more likely to acquire the habit than if neither smoke.

Perhaps as many as one out of three American adults have stopped smoking. This means that anyone can stop if he or she is sufficiently motivated. Unfortunately, often only fear of imminent death causes people to quit. We do not recommend that our patients try to stop smoking and lose weight at the same time; this is impossible for most people. If the diet is not well under control, ten to thirty pounds of weight gain may follow cessation of smoking. If the patient relapses and starts smoking again, he may be thirty pounds heavier and none the better as far as smoking is concerned. Therefore, we recommend that our overweight smokers either work on weight reduction or smoking, but not both at the same time. Some patients stop smoking by going "cold turkey"; some have used a set of progressively restricting filters to reduce the amount of smoke reaching the lungs; some have weaned themselves by such measures as gradually decreasing the number of cigarettes, by laying down the cigarette between puffs, by inhaling few times and less deeply, by putting the cigarette out before it is smoked to the end and by choosing a brand with a low nicotine and tar content; other patients have entered programs that use behavior modification techniques. Whichever method is employed we cannot emphasize too strongly the perils of the smoking habit to general health.

Secondary Risk Factors

Diabetes Mellitus. Diabetes mellitus is defined as an abnormal elevation of blood sugar, of *hyperglycemia,* one of the most important secondary risk factors for atherosclerosis. In addition to the usual varieties of large vessel atherosclerosis, diabetics also suffer from a disease involving the small blood vessels. The decrease in risk of coronary heart disease for the premenopausal female is canceled by the presence of diabetes.

One pathological characteristic of diabetes is the thickening of the basement membrane structure just outside the endothelial layer of blood vessels. There is disagreement as to whether this abnormality precedes the onset of hyperglycemia or whether it is a secondary phenomenon.

The definition of diabetes mellitus is somewhat tenuous at the present time. Diabetes is usually diagnosed on the basis of an elevation of the blood sugar at a given length of time after administration of an oral dose of sugar. The American Diabetes Association has published a normal range of values for glucose tolerance tests. There is a popular misconception that diabetes is caused by eating too much sugar; this is not true. The level of the blood sugar, or glucose, is regulated largely by hormones, among which two of the most important are insulin and glucagon. These two hormones are produced by the pancreas, a six-inch-long gland located near the stomach. Glucagon causes an elevation of blood glucose through glycogen breakdown by the liver; insulin causes a decrease in blood sugar by stimulating the uptake of glucose into cells and tissues. The ratio of glucagon to insulin is an important factor in determining the level of blood glucose.

There are two general types of diabetes: juvenile, or insulin-dependent, and adult-onset. In the juvenile-type diabetes, which may not occur until adulthood, there is usually a severe deficiency or a complete absence of insulin. The isolation of insulin revolutionized the treatment of this disorder. Prior to the use of insulin, the life expectancy of a child after the onset of diabetes was measured in weeks or months. Now, the average life expectancy of an insulin-dependent diabetic is approximately thirty years after the onset of the disease. Diabetics appear to be more susceptible to infection than normal individuals, and the discovery and introduction of antibiotics has contributed to an increase in the longevity of patients with this disease. The treatment for the juvenile diabetic is insulin, diet and exercise. The diet should be a balanced one containing approximately 40 to 45 percent of the calories as carbohydrates, 35 to 40 percent as fat, and 20 percent as protein. While there is restriction of free sugar, or sucrose, the main purpose of the diet is to achieve normal growth and development in the child. An excessive restriction of carbohydrates is no longer recommended. Exercise helps to burn up blood sugar and may decrease the amount of insulin required to regulate the diabetic. There is an increased metabolism of glucose by skeletal muscle during exercise, even in the face of a low level of circulating insulin.

Adult-onset diabetes is usually less severe than the juvenile disease. Some adult diabetics may actually secrete too much insulin prior to developing overt diabetes. The adult-onset diabetic usually is able to secrete some insulin, although there may be a relative deficiency of the hormone. The primary treatment of adult-onset diabetes is weight control, diet, and exercise.

For a number of years oral agents have been used in the treatment of adult-onset diabetes. Some of these drugs, such as tolbutamide, increase the secretion of insulin by the pancreas. A great deal of controversy exists today over use of oral agents for the treatment of diabetes. One controversial study claimed that they may actually increase the death rate from coronary artery disease. Accordingly, the use of oral agents to lower blood sugar should be instituted only as a last resort, i.e., if the measures of weight control, diet and exercise fail.

The occurrence of diabetes does not mean that the affected individual cannot live an active life. One has only to look at the achievements of Bill Talbert in tennis, Ham Richardson, Rhodes Scholar and tennis star, Ron Santo, former third baseman for the Chicago Cubs, and of actress and dancer Mary Tyler Moore to illustrate this point.

It is not yet known whether strict control of the blood sugar by the diabetic will prevent the onset of cardiovascular complications. Atherosclerosis, blindness, kidney failure, and neuropathy are the major clinical complications that diabetics must face. Actually, the blood sugar level is not very closely regulated in most diabetics. It will probably be a number of years before we are able to determine whether or not strict control of the blood sugar in diabetics will prevent or retard the development of vascular and other complications.

In 1976, the American Diabetes Association took the position, enunciated by its president, Dr. George Cahill, that normalization of the blood sugar should be the objective of diabetic control and that there is now evidence that such control will lessen the likelihood of vascular complications. In order to try to maintain the diabetic's level of blood sugar as close as possible to the normal range, multiple daily injections of insulin are required. This form of treatment carries a danger of giving too much insulin and causing hypoglycemia, or low blood sugar. Hypoglycemia is usually associated with weakness and sweating and may lead to loss of consciousness and damage to the central nervous system.

We recommend an approach of moderation. Excessive hyperglycemia, for example, to the extent that thirst and overproduction of urine occur, should be avoided as should hypoglycemia. The degree of diabetic control varies with each individual patient. It is our hope that more effective means of regulating blood sugar will be developed because only then will we be able to obtain a definitive answer about the protection provided by close control of the blood sugar.

A number of important advances in the field of diabetes research may occur in the next few years, including the development of devices for minute-to-minute control of the blood sugar, transplantation of pancreatic tissue and treatment of nerve cell damage.

Obesity and Diet. Obesity directly or indirectly may affect a number of the coronary artery disease risk factors. For example, it tends to exacerbate hypertension, to elevate triglycerides, and it certainly worsens glucose tolerance and diabetes. There may also be a relationship between obesity and a lack of physical activity. In the Framingham study referred to earlier, it was found that there is a very strong relationship between an increase in body weight and angina pectoris, myocardial infarction, and sudden death. This correlation is stronger in men than in women. If you think about it, the excess fat imposes an additional burden on the heart by requiring more oxygen from the bloodstream. Life expectancy statistics have long shown a higher mortality from cardiovascular disease in overweight individuals. For most people, the ideal body weight is close to what they weighed at age 21, provided that they were not already overweight at that time. As individuals grow older and physical activity decreases, calories pile up as excess body fat. Obesity is one of the plagues of an affluent society. There is overwhelming epidemiological evidence to support the fact that during periods of relative starvation in the Second World War, the incidence of coronary artery disease in Europe and the Soviet Union fell to virtually zero.

While starvation is not required in our society, some degree of moderation is. Calories do count and if the daily intake of calories is reduced below the daily use of calories, weight reduction will certainly result. We do not recommend a crash or fad diet, which can be quite dangerous, especially for patients with diabetes, kidney or liver disease. For example, a high fat diet can lead to an increase in the serum cholesterol. Any weight-loss program that changes the normal eating habits should not be taken without the guidance of a physician.

We recommend that individuals lose weight by following a balanced diet with fewer calories. During the period of caloric restriction, you should learn the principles of the diet that you will follow after you have lost the desired amount of weight and are placed on a maintenance diet. Losing the pounds is only half the story. The real challenge is in maintaining the weight reduction over the succeeding weeks, months and years. It is for this reason that gradual reduction is recommended and why crash diets are notoriously unsuccessful in the long run.

Exercise. One of the first points to be made about exercise should be to correct the popular misconception that people who suffer from obesity can reduce simply by increasing their physical exertion. Whether a person loses or gains weight is determined by his daily intake and expenditure of calories. Physical exertion without a regulated diet cannot combat obesity. In order to lose weight an exercise program must be coordinated with a dieting program.

Perhaps we should first discuss just what exercise is and how it is related to the cardiovascular system. One of the questions most frequently asked by patients is, will exercise keep me from having a heart attack and what good will it do me? There is some evidence, largely derived from epidemiological studies, that a high degree of physical activity will prevent heart attacks and atherosclerosis. However, this has not been proven in a scientifically controlled experiment. We agree with the position of the Committee on Exercise of the American Heart Association which stated, "Therefore, we do not consider it justifiable to advocate widespread adoption of vigorous exercise programs purely on the ground that exercise alone will prevent heart disease."

We encourage our patients to exercise regularly, but as with diet, this program must be tailored to ability and individual interests. Such a regular exercise regimen will improve the quality of life by increasing physical ability for work and other activities. For patients who are recuperating from a heart attack, stroke, or cardiovascular surgery, or for those with angina pectoris, controlled physical activity can be an important part of a rehabilitation program. Also, exercise can be used as a supplementary activity to control obesity, blood pressure and serum lipid levels, although it cannot substitute for primary control of the risk factor per se.

It should be pointed out that high-level exercise presents a small risk for some middle-aged adults. Occasionally joggers die while exercising. On the opening day of deer season, there seems to be an increased number of heart attacks among middle-aged hunters. It is our view that a person over forty should have a medical evaluation which includes an exercise electrocardiogram, before undertaking a program of physical exercise. As to the type of the exercise, it may take almost any form, including walking, swimming, cycling, tennis or calisthenics. The sessions need be no more than fifteen to thirty minutes and should be as frequent as three to five times per week. We do stress that the program should be tailored to the interests of the individual and should not be something that is a distasteful chore to carry out. Those unaccustomed to exercise should begin with a very low degree of activity and gradually increase it over a period of weeks.

Personality Type and Stress. Popularized by the book *Type A Personality and Coronary Heart Disease* by Drs. Meyer Friedman and Ray Rosenman, personality type has begun to receive attention as a possible risk factor. It is related to, but different from, stress, another potential risk factor. Sudden emotional or physical stress will elevate the blood pressure and cause the heart to pump against increased resistance. Usually the body makes an appropriate adjustment to the stress, but it is conceivable that chronic stress could have an adverse effect on the cardiovascular system by indirectly affecting a number of the risk factors. In addition to blood pressure, a stressful environment may cause an individual to smoke more, to eat more and gain weight, and to follow an improper diet. The so-called Type A personality is the hard-driving person who creates stressful circumstances even where they do not exist; he never relaxes or takes an afternoon off from work, he paces up and down at the airport waiting for a plane and is constantly conscious of time.

By contrast, the Type B personality takes life more in stride, and according to Friedman and Rosenman, is less prone to heart attacks. Most people do not have a typical Type A or Type B personality, but exhibit features somewhere in between the two extremes. One of the difficulties in evaluating the stress and personality theory of coronary disease is the evaluation of personality types. On theoretical grounds, conditions which result in high levels of the catecholamines, adrenalin and noradrenalin, can have a toxic effect on the heart muscle. Stress and personality type are factors which could potentially alter the secretion of these hormones. Whether they have a significant role in the development of atherosclerosis remains to be established.

In individuals who have preexisting coronary artery disease, emotional and physical stress may precipitate attacks of angina and conceivably might even bring on a heart attack. Or, in individuals with cerebrovascular disease, a stroke or cerebrovascular accident may ensue.

Often our patients who have coronary disease ask us if they should change their jobs or their life styles. There is no universally correct answer to this question. For many individuals the tension and emotional stress is inwardly rather than outwardly generated. For such individuals, there will be emotional stress whatever the situation. There are some instances in which we do recommend that our patients who are placed in conditions of severe stress change their jobs or life styles. This is by no means a blanket recommendation and has to be carefully worked out for each individual patient. A sensible life style combining a proper balance of work, physical and intellectual activity, family and social life and some relaxation is the ideal. But it may not be possible to achieve it in all instances, given the demands that life places on us.

Alcohol. As a food, alcohol provides little nutritive value, just additional calories. An excessive consumption of alcohol, more than two ounces per day, may cause an elevation of blood triglycerides. If someone is overweight or diabetic and is trying to control calories, the consumption of alcohol must be taken into account along with the other food consumed. A small amount of alcohol taken in moderation cannot be shown to have a direct toxic effect on the cardiovascular system in most individuals. However, an excessive consumption of spirits and beer has been associated with a group of disorders in which the heart muscle itself is directly weakened; these are referred to as cardiomyopathies. The heart becomes enlarged and weakened and does not respond well to medical or surgical treatment. Excessive drinking can damage the liver and may lead to certain forms of central nervous system disorders. Alcoholism itself and all of its ramifications is one of the great social plagues on our society today. Moderation is strongly suggested as far as alcohol consumption is concerned.

Uric Acid. A high level of serum uric acid is associated with an increased incidence of arteriosclerosis. There is a correlation between elevations of uric acid, high blood triglycerides and obesity. All of these are made worse by excessive alcohol consumption. There is little evidence that uric acid per se, apart from its association with hypertriglyceridemia, is a direct risk factor for coronary disease. In cardiac patients, an elevation of uric acid may occur in susceptible individuals who are treated with thiazide diuretics. Control of alcohol intake, weight and triglycerides often will decrease the elevation of uric acid. Prolonged *hyperuricemia* may eventually lead to kidney damage. In the presence of primary hyperuricemia, a serum uric acid of over 9 milligrams percent requires medical attention and should be treated.

Sex. There are a number of risk factors over which the patient has no control. One of these, of course, is whether we are male or female. It is a well-established fact that women are protected against atherosclerosis prior to menopause and, statistically, the risk of coronary heart disease death is lower than for men. When risk factors are present in women, they certainly should be treated. We have seen many young women with hyperlipidemia, diabetes mellitus or hypertension who have severe coronary artery disease by their late twenties or thirties. Between ages forty and forty-nine the incidence of clinically significant coronary artery disease in men is about five times greater than in women. Above age fifty, the ratio begins to decrease.

The reasons for the protection against atherosclerosis in premenopausal females are not known. Probably, the effect is related to production of the female sex hormone, estrogen, which declines after menopause. Unfortunately, there is no evidence that treatment with estrogen will protect against heart attacks. There is good evidence that men should not be treated with estrogens. In the first place, large doses of estrogen produce unacceptable, feminizing side effects. In the Coronary Drug Project* completed in 1975, men who had had one or more heart attacks were treated with 2.5 or 5.0 milligrams of estrogen; there was a higher incidence of new heart attacks, pulmonary emboli and overall mortality in the groups receiving estrogen treatment. Thus at the present time, estrogen therapy has no place in the treatment of coronary artery disease.

Heredity. Heredity plays a major part in determining an individual's susceptibility to coronary artery disease. Obviously, this is another risk factor over which the individual has no control. There are genetic susceptibilities to elevation of cholesterol and triglycerides, hypertension, obesity and perhaps even to coronary artery disease and arteriosclerosis in ways we do not yet know.

To sum up, preventive maintenance begins with a complete medical evaluation and with a program to reduce known risk factors. One of the keys

---

*This was a study of over 8,000 male survivors of heart attacks sponsored by the National Heart and Lung Institute in fifty-three American centers.

to reducing the risk certainly is a well-planned diet, and another is the avoidance of cigarette smoking. If hyperlipidemia, diabetes, obesity or hypertension are present, they should be treated. The life style should be balanced with some physical activity and moderation in the consumption of food and alcoholic beverages. For the average person, moderation in all phases of life becomes the cardiovascular system as well as serenity.

GLOSSARY

Acidosis—A metabolic condition in which the acid content of the blood or body tissues is too great; acidosis may result from failure of the lungs to remove carbon dioxide or from an overproduction of acid substances in the body's tissues; the former is called respiratory acidosis and the latter, metabolic acidosis.

Adipose tissue—Fat cells or fat tissues of the body.

Adrenal cortex—The outer, firm, yellowish layer that comprises the larger part of the adrenal gland where hormones of the "cortisol" family are produced.

Adrenal medulla—The innermost part of the adrenal gland; secretes adrenalin and noradrenalin.

Adrenalin—Synonymous with epinephrine; a hormone secreted by the adrenal medulla which has profound effects on blood vessels, the heart and the bronchioles in the lungs. The hormone's actions on the heart, arterioles and bronchioles have been classified as alpha and beta. The beta effects, which may be shown at relatively low dosages, include relaxing the smooth muscles of the arterioles and bronchioles but stimulating the rate and contraction force of the heart. At higher concentrations the alpha actions predominate, especially the contraction of arterioles, leading to a rise in blood pressure.

ADVENTITIA—The outermost layer of the arterial wall; rich in connective tissue and nerve fibers; contains a specialized group of blood vessels called vasa vasorum.

ALBUMIN—A protein made by the liver and transported in the blood; it helps to maintain the fluid within the vascular tree and transports fatty acids.

ALDOSTERONE—The principle electrolyte regulating steroid secreted by the cortex of the adrenal gland.

ALPHAMETHYLDOPA—An orally effective hypotensive agent related to the cate-cholamines; used in the treatment of essential hypertension.

ALVEOLI—Small air sacs in the lung from which blood receives oxygen and gives off carbon dioxide.

AMYLOID—A protein structure which may collect in tissues in certain diseases.

ANABOLISM—Those metabolic reactions in which cells or tissues and large molecules are synthesized or built up.

ANAEROBIC REACTIONS—A reaction which takes place in the absence of oxygen.

ANASTOMOSIS—A connection between vessels and/or grafts.

ANGIOGRAPHY—The study of blood vessels, either arteries or veins, made by the injection of a radiopaque substance, permitting visualization by x-ray.

ANEURYSM—Balloonlike sac formed by the dilatation of the walls of an artery damaged by arteriosclerosis.

ANGINA PECTORIS—Spasmodic chest pains usually resulting from decreased blood flow to the heart caused by atherosclerotic disease of the coronary arteries.

ANGIOTENSIN II—A vasoconstrictor substance present in the blood and formed by the action of renin on a globulin of the blood plasma.

ANOXIA—The condition in which there is the absence of oxygen.

AORTA—The main artery carrying blood from the heart to the rest of the body. The ascending aorta is that part between the heart and the aortic arch where it turns to become the descending aorta; the aorta within the chest or thorax is known as the thoracic aorta and within the abdomen is called the abdominal aorta.

AORTIC ARCH—The point in the aorta at which it curves from an upward to a downward direction within the chest or thoracic cavity.

ARRHYTHMIA—Any variation from the normal rhythm of the heartbeat.

ARTERIAL THROMBOSIS—A blood clot formed within the arterial system; this is the type of thrombosis that can cause heart attacks and strokes; it is rich in blood platelets and is sometimes called a "white" thrombosis because of its appearance.

ARTERIOGRAM—X-ray picture of the lumen or channel of an artery made by injecting a radiopaque substance into the blood (see RADIOPAQUE).

ARTERIOLES—Small muscular vessels that are formed from the small branches of arteries; the arterioles then branch to form the capillaries.

ARTERIOSCLEROSIS—Disease of arteries, often referred to as hardening of the arteries. It includes and is often used synonymously with atherosclerosis. While the latter term refers primarily to disease of intima, arteriosclerosis may also include disease of the arterial media.

ARTERY—A vessel that carries blood from the heart to the tissues of the body, ending in small branches called arterioles which in turn branch to form the capillaries.

ASYMPTOMATIC—Showing or causing no symptoms.

ATHEROMA—See ATHEROMATOUS PLAQUE.

ATHEROMATOUS PLAQUE (ATHEROMA)—A focal deposition of lipid, or fatty material, and cholesterol within the intimal layer of the artery, which may progress to narrow or block the lumen of an artery and is the most common cause of heart attacks and strokes.

ATHEROSCLEROSIS—A form of arteriosclerosis in which there is a characteristic focal deposition of lipids initially within the intimal layer of the artery; associated with a growth of smooth muscle cells and other changes in the arterial wall; this form of arteriosclerosis causes most strokes and heart attacks.

ATHEROSCLEROTIC CORONARY ARTERY DISEASE—A form of hardening of the arteries in which cholesterol and lipid accumulate within the arterial wall of the coronary arteries at first affecting primarily the intimal layer of the artery and leading to narrowing or occlusion of the vessel.

ATRIAL FIBRILLATION—A type of heart irregularity in which the atrial contractions are poor and irregular, and not coordinated with those of the ventricle.

ATRIAL SEPTAL DEFECT—A common type of heart defect in which there is a hole in the septum or wall between the left and right atria.

ATRIOVENTRICULAR NODE—The specialized bundle of muscle and nerve tissue located in the wall of the right ventricle; it is stimulated by impulses from the sinoatrial node to discharge impulses that result in contraction of the heart muscle.

ATRIUM—The small antechambers of the heart which receive blood from the lungs and body.

ATROPHY—The wasting away or diminution in size of a tissue or cell.

ATP—Abbreviation for adenosine triphosphate—a chemical compound present in all cells representing a storage form of energy.

BACTERIAL ENDOCARDITIS—A bacterial infection or inflammation of the inner lining of the heart affecting the heart valves (often valves previously damaged by, for example, rheumatic fever).

BALL VALVE PRINCIPLE—Consists of a ball that fits in a cage over a cup-shaped opening in the seat. As the ball rises in the cage, fluid or air escapes through the opening in the seat, and as the ball falls into the seat, the valve closes, preventing the escaped material from passing back through the opening.

BARORECEPTORS—Specialized sensory nerve endings sensitive to changes in blood pressure located at certain sites in the walls of arteries, such as the aortic arch and carotid sinus, which is at or above the bifurcation of the carotid arteries in the neck; they are sensitive to changes in pressure and function to maintain the blood pressure within the "normal range."

BASEMENT MEMBRANE—The delicate layer of extracellular condensation of the chemical substances mucopolysaccharides and proteins underlying the epithelium of mucous membranes and outside the endothelium of blood vessels; diabetics develop a thickening of the basement membrane of blood vessels in smooth muscle cells and in the kidneys.

BIFURCATION—Division into two branches.

BLALOCK–TAUSSIG OPERATION—A surgical procedure developed by Dr. Alford Blalock and Dr. Helen Taussig at The Johns Hopkins School of Medicine for the treatment of the congenital heart defect tetralogy of Fallot; consists of creating an artificial shunt from a nearby artery to the pulmonary artery in order to bypass the narrowed, stenotic pulmonary valve.

BLOOD GROUPS—A system of classification based on the presence of substances called agglutinogens on human red blood cells and antibodies to these substances in the serum. The major blood groups in man are A, B, AB and O. Red blood cells contain agglutinogen, A (group A), B (group B), A plus B (group AB) or neither (group O). An individual's serum contains antibodies to the agglutinogen(s) not present on his red blood cells. There are other subgroups and additional markers besides these major ones.

BLOOD LETTING—The removal of blood from a vein, once used as a form of treatment for many types of disease.

BLOOD TRANSFUSION—The removal of blood from the vein of one person (donor) and its intravenous administration into the vein of another individual (recipient).

BRUIT—A murmur; a swishing noise produced by the blood as it rushes through an artery narrowed by an obstructive lesion.

BYPASS OPERATION—A surgical procedure in which a graft is attached to an artery above and below the site of obstruction for the purpose of providing a normal blood flow distal to the diseased vessel.

CALCIFICATION—The process by which tissues, including those of the arterial wall, become hardened by a deposit of calcium.

CALCIUM DEPOSITION—See CALCIFICATION.

CANNULA—A tube used for insertion into a blood vessel or the heart.

CANNULATE—To pass a cannula or tube into the heart or a blood vessel.

CAPILLARIES—Small vessels, only one cell in thickness, from which blood supplies oxygen and nutrients to tissues; formed by the branching of arterioles, they combine into larger vessels called venules.

CARDIAC TAMPONADE—A condition usually caused by bleeding from the heart or a major vessel near the heart that rapidly fills the pericardial sac around the heart with blood, resulting in compression of the heart; usually produces death in a very short time unless corrected by removing the blood or fluid.

CARDIOMYOPATHY—A group of diseases often of undetermined cause characterized by dysfunction of the heart muscle and by heart failure due to weakness and dysfunction of the heart muscle cells per se; other causes of heart failure must be excluded.

CARDIOPULMONARY BYPASS—Used synonymously with heart-lung machine; venous blood is diverted to the artificial lung of the machine where it is oxygenated and carbon dioxide is removed; the oxygenated blood is pumped back into the patient's arterial system.

CARDIOVASCULAR SYPHILIS—Syphilis affects the cardiovascular system many years after the primary infection; the aortic valve ring may become dilated producing aortic insufficiency and there may be pathological changes in the wall of the aorta that may lead to aneurysm.

CAROTID ARTERIES—The principal arteries which supply blood to the brain; they arise from the innominate artery on the right and the arch of the aorta on the left.

CAROTID SINUS—A bulblike structure at or above the bifurcation of the common carotid artery into the external and internal carotid arteries in the neck. The sinus, which is in the wall of the artery, contains specialized nerve endings that respond to distention of the wall produced by a rise in blood pressure. These receptors function to maintain normal blood pressure.

CATABOLISM—Those metabolic reactions in which cells or tissues and large molecules are broken down.

CATECHOLAMINE—A group of compounds that contain the structure catechol to which a portion containing an amine is attached; adrenalin or epinephrine, noradrenalin, or norepinephrine and dopamine are examples; they exert actions on the cardiovascular system associated with the sympathetic nervous system.

CELIAC ARTERY—An artery that arises from the abdominal aorta and divides into arteries supplying blood to the liver, spleen and stomach.

CEREBELLUM—One of the divisions of the brain; concerned with the coordination of movements.

CEREBROVASCULAR—Pertaining to the blood vessels of the cerebrum or brain.

CHOLESTEROL—Type of animal fat called a sterol; the body gets cholesterol both by making it, and from the diet.

CHORDAE TENDINAE—Stringlike attachments that connect the edges of the mitral and tricuspid valves to the papillary muscles in the ventricles of the heart; they resemble ropes attached to the edges of a parachute.

CHOREA—Disorder of the central nervous system which is characterized by spastic twitchings of the muscles.

CIRCLE OF WILLIS—A network of arteries resembling a circle; formed by the main arteries supplying the brain, located at the base of the brain.

CIRCUMFLEX CORONARY ARTERY—One of the two main branches that normally originates from the left coronary artery; supplies blood to the left lateral and posterior aspects of the heart.

COARCTATION OF THE AORTA—A congenital heart defect in which there is a severe narrowing of the aorta, usually in the distal part of the arch.

COLLAGEN TISSUE—A type of fibrous connective protein tissue that supports the skin, tendons, arterial wall, etc.

COLLATERAL CIRCULATION—The development of connections around an obstruction to blood flow through the growth of small arteries above and below the obstruction; nature's method of compensating for an obstruction in blood flow.

CONGENITAL CORONARY ARTERY DISEASE—A form of inherited abnormality in the coronary arteries.

CONTRACTILITY OF THE HEART—The ability of the heart muscle to contract and pump blood.

CORONARY ARTERIOGRAPHY—A study of the coronary arteries performed by introducing a catheter to inject radiopaque dye which permits visualization of the vessels by x-rays.

CYANOSIS—A clinical condition characterized by a bluish appearance caused by a lack of oxygen in the blood.

CYSTIC MEDIAL NECROSIS—Death of cells in media of the arterial wall, with the formation of a cyst or open space at the site of tissue destruction; this condition may lead to a dissection of the layers of the artery's wall, a catastrophic cardiovascular situation.

DIASTOLE—The phase of the heart's cycle during which it relaxes and fills its chambers with blood.

DIGITALIS—A drug which when administered in the proper dosage stimulates the contractility and slows the failing heart; an excess of digitalis can result in poisoning and produce severe toxicity.

DISTAL—Remote, farther from any point of reference; opposite of proximal.

DIURETIC—An agent that promotes the excretion of urine.

DUCTUS ARTERIOSUS—The fetal blood vessel that connects the pulmonary artery with the aorta; in some cases may fail to close at birth resulting in the congenital abnormality of patent ductus arteriosus.

DUCTUS VENOSUS—A vessel that brings oxygenated blood from the mother's placenta to the fetus; this vessel bypasses the liver of the fetus and goes directly to the right atrium.

EDEMA—The presence of abnormally large amounts of fluid in the intracellular tissue spaces of the body.

ELASTIN—A type of elastic tissue which occurs in the wall of arteries and other tissues of the body.

ELECTROCARDIOGRAM—A recording of a tracing of the heart's electrical activities, usually measured in a standard way.

ELECTROCARDIOGRAPHY—Recording of the electrical impulses of the heart, usually in the form of the electrocardiogram.

EMBOLECTOMY—An operation in which an embolus (see below) is removed from a blood vessel.

EMBOLUS—A clot or other matter which travels through the bloodstream to lodge in a small vessel and cause an obstruction to the circulation.

EMPHYSEMA—The loss of elasticity of the bronchi in the lungs resulting in a chronic overexpansion in the lungs leading to shortness of breath.

ENCEPHALOPATHY—Any degenerative disease of the brain.

ENDARTERECTOMY—A surgical procedure in which an artery is opened and the atherosclerotic lesion is peeled away from the arterial wall and removed; the incision may be closed by suturing of the remaining normal walls, or with a patch graft which provides for a widely patent lumen in the previously diseased vessel.

ENDOCARDIAL FIBROELASTOSIS—A condition in which there is an overgrowth of the endocardium or lining of the left ventricle, resulting in a thickening that decreases the volume capacity of the left ventricle.

ENDOCARDIUM—The inner lining of the heart which is in contact with the blood.

ENDOTHELIUM—The innermost layer of cells lining a blood vessel.

EPICARDIUM—The outer layer of the heart in contact with the pericardial sac which contains the heart.

ERYTHROCYTES—The red blood cells containing hemoglobin; their main function being the transport of oxygen.

ESTERS—Chemical compounds that are formed from an alcohol and an acid by the removal of water.

ETIOLOGY—The study of the cause of any disease.

EXCISION—The surgical removal of a diseased segment of tissue or vessel.

EXSANGUINATION—Forceful expulsion of blood from the body.

EXTRACELLULAR—Outside of a cell or cells.

EXTRACORPOREAL CIRCULATION—Circulation of the blood through a mechanical device, usually a heart-lung machine, outside the patient's body.

EXTRACRANIAL ARTERIES—Arteries supplying blood to the brain before they enter the skull.

FEMORAL ARTERY—An artery in the upper leg.

FIBRIN—An elastic filament protein that is formed by the action of thrombin to produce the clotting of blood.

FIBRINOGEN—A long fibrillar protein found in the blood; transformed to a smaller protein called fibrin during the formation of a blood clot.

FIBROMUSCULAR HYPERPLASIA—The abnormal increase in the number of normal muscle cells in an artery causing thickening of the wall and narrowing or occlusion of the vessel; most frequently it occurs in the renal arteries, where it may cause hypertension.

FIBROSIS—The formation of fibrous tissue.

FIBROUS PLAQUE—A type of atherosclerotic lesion which is covered by a cap of fibrous tissue containing collagen, elastic fibers and smooth muscle cells filled with fat; most of the total fat in the plaque is found outside the cells, however.

FORAMEN OVALE—An oval opening in the septum of the fetal heart between the right and left atrium that normally closes after birth.

FUSIFORM—Spindle-shaped.

GANGLIA—Knotlike masses of a group of nerve cell bodies located outside the central nervous system.

GLOBULINS—A group of blood proteins, some of which function as antibodies.

GLYCOGEN—Chemically a polysaccharide that is formed and stored in the liver, muscles and, to a lesser extent, in other tissues. It is the chief carbohydrate storage material in the body and is readily converted into glucose when needed.

HEMOGLOBIN—A conjugated protein within the red blood cells (erythrocytes) that is capable of transporting oxygen and carbon dioxide.

HEPARIN—A mucopolysaccharide acid occuring in various tissues, but most abundantly in the liver; when injected into the circulation it blocks blood coagulation and promotes the clearing of triglyceride fat.

HETEROGRAFT—Nonhuman animal tissue used to replace a diseased blood vessel or organ.

HOMEOSTASIS—A state of equilibrium in which the chemical substances and various components of the body are in balance with each other.

HOMOGRAFT—Human tissue used to replace a diseased blood vessel or organ, usually obtained from a cadaver.

HYDROLYZE—To cleave or break a chemical bond with water; for example, a triglyceride is hydrolyzed or broken down into glycerol and free fatty-acid components.

HYPERCHOLESTEROLEMIA—An elevation of the plasma or serum cholesterol concentration.

HYPERLIPIDEMIA—An abnormally high concentration of lipids or fats in the blood.

HYPERLIPIDEMIC SERUM—Serum that contains an elevated concentration of the blood lipids; most often used to refer to serum in which the triglyceride blood fats are elevated.

HYPERTENSION—The condition in which the blood pressure within the arteries is elevated.

HYPERTRIGLYCERIDEMIA—An elevation of the concentration of the plasma or serum triglycerides.

HYPOTHERMIA—The use of low body temperature to reduce cardiac output, pulse rate, blood pressure and oxygen consumption since cells survive longer when chilled.

HYPERTROPHIED MUSCLE—Muscle that is increased in size due to increased activity.

HYPERTROPHY—Enlargement or overgrowth of an organ or body part.

HYPOTHYROIDISM—A thyroid deficiency of thyroid hormones.

HYPOXIA—The condition in which the oxygen level of the body or a tissue is too low.

ILIAC ARTERIES—The terminal branches of the abdominal aorta; the principal arteries supplying blood to the pelvic or hip region and the legs.

ILIOFEMORAL ARTERIES—Pertaining to the iliac and femoral arteries.

INFERIOR MESENTERIC ARTERY—The artery from the abdominal aorta that supplies the lower part of the large intestine.

INFERIOR VENA CAVA—The main vein returning blood to the heart from the lower part of the body.

INNERVATION—The supply of nerves to a part of the body.

INNOMINATE ARTERY—The first of three major arteries which arise from the aortic arch; it divides into the right subclavian and right common carotid arteries.

INTERMITTENT CLAUDICATION—A symptom of arterial occlusive disease in the legs; it is characterized by pain when walking or exercising and by relief of pain on resting.

INTERSTITIAL FLUID—The fluid in which the individual cells of the body are bathed.

INTIMA—The innermost layer of the arterial wall which is in contact with the blood.

INTRACRANIAL ARTERIES—Arteries within the skull.

ISCHEMIC—The state in which a cell or tissue has an insufficient supply of oxygen.

LEFT ANTERIOR DESCENDING CORONARY ARTERY—One of the two main branches that normally originates from the left coronary artery; supplies blood to the anterior wall of the heart.

LESION—An abnormality in any structure of the body.

LEUKOCYTES—The white blood cells; their main function is to protect the body against infection; there are several different major types, the polymorphonuclear leukocytes, the lymphocytes and the monocytes.

LIPIDS—Fatty substances, including cholesterol, triglyceride and phospholipid, that are present in the blood and in tissues.

LIPOPROTEINS, PLASMA—Macromolecular complexes of lipid and protein that transport all of the plasma lipids or fats, including cholesterol, triglyceride and phospholipid.

LUMBAR SYMPATHECTOMY—Surgical procedure consisting of the excision of a small segment of the lumbar sympathetic nerve ganglia to interrupt the nerve impulses to the muscles in the walls of the arteries of the legs; its purpose is to permit dilation of the smaller arteries and thus to increase blood flow and to allow a greater degree of collateral circulation in the lower leg.

LUMEN—The opening or channel of a blood vessel or other structure.

LYMPHOCYTE—A type of white blood cell involved in antibody reactions; it is produced in lymphoid tissue that constitutes 20 to 30 percent of the white blood cells, or leukocytes, of normal human blood.

MARFAN'S SYNDROME—A group of multiple congenital abnormalities involving connective tissue, often occuring in conjunction with cystic medial necrosis of the aorta; patients with this syndrome generally are very tall with unusually long bones of the arms, legs, feet and hands.

MEDIA—The middle, or muscular, layer of the arterial wall; the media contains smooth muscle cells, elastic tissue and collagen.

MEMBRANE OXYGENATOR—A device made of flat bags of cellophane or Teflon, used to oxygenate blood; a component of the heart-lung machine.

MESENTERIC ARTERIES—The major arteries which supply blood to the gastrointestinal tract.

METABOLISM—The body's chemical processes; metabolic processes are divided into anabolic and catabolic.

MITOCHONDRIA—Specialized structures within the cell which function for the oxidation of food substances and the production of energy.

MITRAL REGURGITATION—Dysfunction of the mitral valve produced when the valve is incompetent or "leaky" and in which blood flows back into the left atrium during systole, the phase in which the heart contracts.

MITRAL VALVE—The valve separating the left atrium from the left ventricle of the heart; also called the bicuspid valve because it is made up of two cusps.

MONOCYTE—A type of white blood cell that is believed to interact with lymphocytes in immune reactions.

MONOGLYCERIDE—A glycerol molecule to which only one fatty acid molecule is attached.

MORPHOLOGICAL—Pertaining to the science of forms and structure of organized beings.

MURAL THROMBUS—A blood clot attached to a diseased part of the inner lining of the heart wall.

MYOCARDIAL INFARCTION—Used synonymously with heart attack or coronary thrombosis, but refers specifically to the death of part of the heart muscle or myocardium; diagnosis is established by clinical manifestations, changes in the electrocardiogram and by measurement of blood enzymes released from the damaged heart muscle.

MYCARDIUM—The muscular tissue of the heart.

MYCOTIC ANEURYSM—An aneurysm produced by lodging of an infected embolus in the vessel's wall.

NEPHRITIS—Inflammation of the kidneys.

NERVE—A structure in the form of a fiber that transmits impulses between the central nervous system and parts of the body.

NEUROPATHY—A general term describing dysfunction and/or pathological changes in the peripheral nervous system.

NITROGLYCERINE—A drug used for many years to treat angina pectoris; usually provides a rapid relief of chest pain within one to three minutes in a patient suffering an attack of angina pectoris.

NONINVASIVE PROCEDURE—A procedure which does not involve injection or insertion of foreign chemicals, catheters or other substances into the patient.

NORADRENALIN—Synonymous with norepinephrine; a hormone secreted by the adrenal medulla which has profound effects on blood vessels, the heart and the entire cardiovascular system; causes the arterioles to contract and the heart rate to increase.

PACEMAKER—The sinoatrial node; a small bundle of muscle fibers and nerves within the right atrium which sends out electrical impulses at regular intervals to cause contraction of the heart.

PACEMAKER, ARTIFICAL—A mechanical device that can be used to control the heart rate and take the place of the patient's own natural pacemaker.

PALLIATIVE—Treatment that provides relief for the condition, but not a cure.

PAPILLARY MUSCLES—The muscles inside the ventricles of the heart which are attached to the mitral and tricuspid valves by means of the chorda tendinae.

PARASYMPATHETIC—Pertaining to one of the two divisions of the autonomic nervous system; parasympathetic activity tends to slow the heart rate and cause a widening or dilation of arterioles.

PATENT DUCTUS ARTERIOSUS—A congenital anomaly consisting of a persistently open lumen of the fetal vessel (ductus arteriosus) between the aorta and pulmonary artery after birth.

PATCH-GRAFT ANGIOPLASTY—A surgical procedure which consists of suturing a patch into an incision in the wall of an artery in order to widen the lumen of the vessel.

PEPTIDE—One of a class of compounds of low molecular weight that contains two or more amino acids; may be formed by the breakdown of proteins or by linking together two or more amino acids; when a peptide reaches a certain, arbitrary size, it becomes known as a protein.

PERICARDIECTOMY—Surgical procedure which consists of stripping off a section of the pericardium, the sac which contains the heart.

PERICARDIAL—Pertaining to the fibroserous sac that contains the heart.

PERICARDITIS—Inflammation of the pericardial sac.

PERICARDIUM—The saclike covering which contains the heart.

PERIPHERAL EMBOLIZATION—Obstruction or occlusion of a distal artery in the limbs, brain or kidney, usually by a clot, but sometimes by a mass of bacteria or other matter transported in the bloodstream from some proximal or central source.

PHEOCHROMOCYTOMA—A tumor derived from cells in the medulla of the adrenal gland or from similar tissue growing outside the gland; characterized by the secretion of adrenal hormones, adrenalin and noradrenalin resulting in high blood pressure.

PHOSPHOLIPID—A lipid or fatty constituent of the blood and of cell membranes containing glycerol, two fatty acids and a phorphorus containing component; essential for the structure of the cell membrane. In the blood it probably functions to keep the cholesterol and triglyceride in solution.

PLAQUE—A well-demarcated area, raised patch or swelling on a body surface. Atheromatous plaques occur on the inner surface of an artery and have a yellowish color produced by fatty deposits.

PLASMA—The fluid part of the blood.

PLASMA LIPOPROTEINS—A macromolecular complex or fat or lipid and protein. The lipoproteins are the vehicle by which fats or lipids are solubilized and transported in the blood.

PLATELET—A cellular element of the blood which may participate in the clotting, or coagulation, mechanism.

PNEUMATIC CUFF A cuff inflated with air used to constrict the artery in the arm in the measurement of blood pressure.

POLYMORPHONUCLEAR LEUKOCYTE—A type of white cell from the blood involved in the protection of the body against infection through ingestion of bacteria.

POLYUNSATURATED FATS—Fats that do not harden at room temperature; usually liquid oils of vegetable origin.

POPLITEAL ARTERY—An artery behind the knee that carries blood from the femoral artery to the lower leg.

PROPOANOL—A drug that blocks certain actions of the adrenal hormones; it is called a beta-blocking agent and is used to treat angina pectoris and cardiac arrhythmias.

PROSTHETIC DEVICE—An artificial material or device used to take the place of a normal structure that has been removed; in the cardiovascular system, a prosthesis may replace a defective heart valve or a diseased blood vessel.

PROXIMAL—Nearest; closer to any point of reference; as opposed to distal.

P/S RATIO—The ratio of the polyunsaturated to saturated fats in the diet.

PULMONARY ARTERY—The vessel transporting blood from the right ventricle to the lungs; the pulmonary artery contains relatively deoxygenated blood which is replenished with oxygen in the lungs.

PULMONARY EDEMA—A condition associated with heart failure in which the left ventricle of the heart does not pump adequately, causing fluid to accumulate within the lungs.

PULMONARY EMBOLUS—A substance that is carried from a distal part of the vascular tree to the lungs where it is too large to pass through the pulmonary vessels; most frequently, an embolus arises from a blood clot in a vein.

PULMONARY HYPERTENSION—The condition in which the pressure in the pulmonary arteries is increased, and which may lead to thickening and damaging of the walls of the vessels, with a back pressure exerted on blood flow from the right ventricle.

PULMONARY VALVE—The valve between the right ventricle and the pulmonary artery.

PULMONARY VEIN—The vessel carrying blood from the lungs back to the left atrium; the pulmonary veins contain blood which has been oxygenated in the lungs.

PYELOGRAM—An x-ray of the kidney and ureters, usually obtained through the intravenous injection of a radiopaque material.

RADIOPAQUE—The property of blocking x-rays resulting in a light or white appearance on the exposed x-ray film.

RAUWOLFIA—Drugs used to treat hypertension; their name comes from their origin, a genus of tropical trees and shrubs, many species of which have been used in South America, Africa, and Asia, as sources of arrow poisons.

RENAL ARTERIES—Major arteries from the abdominal aorta to the kidneys.

RENIN—An enzyme liberated by the kidney when there is a diminished blood flow to it; renin acts on a blood globulin to cause the formation of angiotensin II, a vasoconstrictor peptide.

RHEUMATIC FEVER—An inflammatory disease that usually follows an infection by a Group A beta-streptococcal organism; it is not an infection itself, but a response to the previous infection, probably on an allergic basis; the heart valves and heart tissue are inflamed and there may be inflammation of the large joints and involvement of the nervous system.

ROENTGENOGRAM—X-ray.

SACCIFORM—Shaped like a sac, bag or pouch.

SAPHENOUS VEINS—The two large superficial veins of the leg.

SATURATED FATS—Fats that harden at room temperature; found in foods of animal origin and in some foods of vegetable origin.

SCLEROSING—The process of obliterating through the formation of extensive scarring.

SEPTICEMIA—Severe bacterial infections of the bloodstream.

SEPTUM—A dividing wall or partition.

SERUM—The fluid part of the blood which remains after a blood clot is formed and removed.

SERUM CHOLESTEROL—The cholesterol contained in the serum (see SERUM and CHOLESTEROL).

SINOATRIAL NODE—Called the pacemaker; a small bundle of muscle fibers and nerves within the wall of the right atrium which sends out electrical impulses at regular intervals to cause contraction of the heart.

SINUS OF VALSALVA—Pouchlike enlargements in the aorta just above the aortic valve.

SUBCLAVIAN ARTERIES—Arteries that supply blood to the upper chest, shoulders and arms; the left subclavian arises from the aorta and the right subclavian from the innominate artery.

SUBCUTANEOUS—Beneath the skin.

SUPERIOR MESENTERIC ARTERY—The artery from the abdominal aorta that supplies the small intestine.

SUPERIOR VENA CAVA—The main vein returning blood to the heart from the upper parts of the body.

SYMPATHETIC—Pertaining to one of the two divisions of the autonomic nervous system; sympathetic activity tends to speed up the heart rate and cause a constriction or narrowing of arterioles.

SYNTHETIC GRAFT—An artificial artery of synthetic material that is used to replace a segment of a diseased artery.

SYSTOLE—The phase of the heart's cycle during which the heart muscle contracts to pump blood to the body.

THORACIC—Pertaining to the chest.

THROMBIN—A protein involved in blood clotting; it promotes the formation of a clot by causing the conversion of fibrinogen to fibrin.

THROMBOENDARTERECTOMY—A surgical procedure which consists of removing a blood clot associated with an atheromatous lesion by dissecting or separating it from the arterial wall; the opening in the artery is repaired by suturing the two edges together or by inserting a patch to widen the arterial lumen.

THROMBUS—A clot in a blood vessel or in one of the cavities of the heart, formed by coagulation of the blood.

TISSUE HYPOXIA—Low oxygen content in a tissue.

TRANSPOSITION OF THE GREAT ARTERIES OR VESSELS—A severe form of congenital heart disease; while the basic abnormality is a transposition of the aorta and the pulmonary artery, there are a number of variations.

TRANSVENOUS—Through a vein.

TRICUSPID ATRESIA—A congenital heart defect in which the tricuspid valve is absent; associated with a small right ventricle and an atrial septal defect.

TRICUSPID VALVE—The valve between the right atrium and right ventricle, so called because it has three cusps.

TRIGLYCERIDE—A fat containing a backbone of glycerol to which fatty acids are attached; it may be of either animal or vegetable origin; it is also manufactured by the body.

TRUNCUS ARTERIOSUS—A form of congenital heart defect in which the pulmonary artery arises from the aorta.

TYPE A PERSONALITY—The hard-driving, time-conscious person, who is thought by some doctors to have an increased risk of developing premature coronary artery disease.

TYPE B PERSONALITY—The relaxed, less compulsive person, who some physicians think has a lower risk of developing coronary artery disease than does the hard-driving Type A personality.

UREMIA—An increase in the concentration of urea and other constituents in the blood normally excreted through the kidney; caused by failure of the kidney; used synonymously with kidney failure.

URIC ACID—A compound excreted in the urine of man that represents the end product from the breakdown of nucleic acids and a group of substances known as purines; elevations of blood uric acid are often found in the disease called gout.

VALVULAR DISEASE—Dysfunction or abnormality of the heart valves.

VASA VASORUM—The network of small vessels within the outer portion of the arterial wall; functions to supply oxygen to the outer wall of medium size and large arteries and veins.

VASCULAR—Pertaining to the blood vessels of the body.

VASCULAR RING—A congenital abnormality of the aortic arch in which a part of the developing arch fails to disappear and may obstruct the esophagus or trachea or both.

VASCULAR TREE—The network of blood vessels that carry blood from the heart to the tissues and back again; it is comprised of arteries, arterioles, capillaries, venules, and veins.

VEIN—A vessel that transports blood from the capillaries in the tissues back to the heart.

VENESECTION—Incision of a vein to remove blood, once used as a form of treatment for many types of disease.

VENTRICLES—The large chambers of the heart from which the blood is propelled out to the lungs and the body.

VENTRICULAR FIBRILLATION—A heart irregularity or arrhythmia in which the heart beats very rapidly but ineffectively, so that blood is not pumped out to supply the body; this condition results in death if not corrected very quickly.

VENTRICULAR SEPTAL DEFECT—A common type of heart defect in which there is a hole in the septum, or wall, between the right and left ventricles.

Venules—Small vessels that carry blood back toward the heart from the capillaries; they combine to form larger vessels called veins.

Vertebral arteries—Two arteries that arise from the right and left subclavian arteries and supply blood to the posterior and basal aspects of the brain.

Viscera—Any large internal organ.

INDEX